DOCTOR ON EVEREST

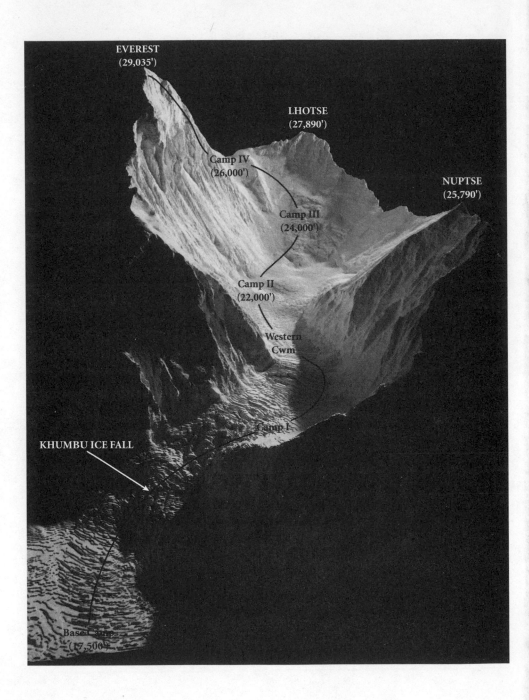

EVEREST
(29,035')

LHOTSE
(27,890')

NUPTSE
(25,790')

Camp IV
(26,000')

Camp III
(24,000')

Camp II
(22,000')

Western
Cwm

Camp I

KHUMBU ICE FALL

Base Camp
(17,500')

DOCTOR ON EVEREST

Emergency Medicine at the Top of the World— A Personal Account Including the 1996 Disaster

Kenneth Kamler, M.D.
with a Foreword by Sir Edmund Hillary

THE LYONS PRESS

Josiane

the wind that fills my sails

FOREWORD

It is nearly fifty years since Tenzing and I first set foot on the summit of Mount Everest and since then a huge number of books have been published about the mountain. But *Doctor on Everest*, written by Dr. Kenneth Kamler, is very different. It describes in great detail the life of one of the most important members of any great challenge—the expedition doctor—who is so frequently overlooked while attention is focussed on the members of the climbing team aiming for the summit.

We are all aware that exploration and climbing have changed dramatically over the past fifty years. In 1953 when we climbed Everest we were fit and strongly motivated but our equipment and food was rather limited. Before us we had a great psychological barrier—we didn't know if it was humanly possible to reach the summit of Everest and survive. This barrier disappeared when Tenzing and I stepped safely on the top of the world.

The modern explorer has greater technical ability and far better equipment. He is able to tackle much harder challenges, such as more dangerous routes and facing climbs and ascents without oxygen. By achieving these more difficult approaches he gains the same satisfaction that we felt in being the first to the summit.

There have been many changes in other ways too. By contributing a large sum of money a relatively inexperienced climber can be conducted by a guide high up the mountain and even to the summit itself. The regular routes are tamed with thousands of meters of fixed rope and scores of aluminum ladders. But Everest remains a difficult and dangerous mountain. Bad weather can stop any climb and the thin air at extreme altitude can sap the energy and even the intelligence of the strongest climber.

So in many ways an expedition doctor has become more and more important. His task is to constantly advise his team on how to safely deal with altitude problems and when an accident occurs, as they often do, it is his responsibility to treat the patient—even in a life-threatening situation. In addition, the expedition doctor is frequently the person the team turns to in moments of stress and danger.

Dr. Kenneth Kamler has been a physician on many Everest expeditions. He has undoubtedly saved many lives and comforted numerous distressed people. He expertly uses modern medicine and techniques to not only deal with common ailments but to also perform life-saving actions in often dangerous and austere conditions.

Ken Kamler played an invaluable role during the disaster on Everest in 1996 when so many died. His description of these days makes a gripping story. I do not believe that on our expedition forty-three years earlier such a devastating experience would ever have occurred—we were too careful, too aware of the weather dangers, and too experienced a team. But things have changed considerably—there are some better climbers on the mountain now and much worse ones too. There is undoubtedly a greater need for highly skilled and equipped doctors like Ken Kamler.

And so we change, sometimes forward and sometimes backward: better equipped and maybe a little more casual. But when the going gets tough and things go wrong, the same qualities are needed to win through as were needed in the past—courage, resourcefulness, the ability to put up with discomfort, and above all, strong motivation. Ken Kamler has shown he possesses all these qualities in full measure.

—Sir Edmund Hillary, 2000

PROLOGUE

I was a little kid when I first became interested in mountain climbing. My first climb was as an eight-year-old when I went up my father's bookshelf and pulled down a book called *Annapurna*. It had such a funny title, I couldn't imagine what it was about. It turned out to be a classic mountaineering tale of the ascent of what was at the time the highest mountain ever climbed. I don't know what my father was doing with that book—no one around me had ever spoken about mountain climbing, much less actually done it—but the book opened up for me, at an impressionable age, a world I never knew existed, impossibly far away from my apartment house in the Bronx. The idea stuck to me and never let go.

It was at about this time that I got my first microscope and discovered another hidden world. Growing up in New York City, it was a lot easier to look through a microscope than to climb a mountain. I had an inclination toward science which my parents were only too eager to encourage, and I enjoyed exploring the natural world—even on a small scale.

My parents' passion was travel, and by the time I was a teenager, I had been all over North America and Europe. This was in the days when most people had never been on an airplane and a trip to Florida was considered pushing the limits. Friends were in awe when I told them I had been to

Paris and London. The usual response was "Wow, you've been everywhere!" It occurred to me even then that actually I had hardly been anywhere. There were so many hidden corners, not to mention whole continents, that I hadn't yet seen. As I got a little older, traveling with my parents suddenly wasn't "cool" anymore. We were going to ever more exotic countries, but if the sights were listed in a guidebook they lost their appeal for me. It was the secret places I didn't want to miss out on.

The combination of science and nature led me into biology and then into the exploration of nature's ultimate secret place, the human body. I became a doctor. My microscope was never forgotten and, like an old friend, it came back to me later as I learned to be a microsurgeon.

Mountain climbing was never forgotten either, although for a long time it remained suspended like a mist in the back of my mind. Climbing was remote—something for people in a different life.

ACKNOWLEDGMENTS

Writing this book was a joyful adventure from beginning to end, though at times it seemed climbing Mount Everest might be easier. Like many expeditions, it required the blending of talented people form several different worlds.

In the literary world, first and foremost, I must say thank you to my agent and fellow explorer, Lindley Kirksey, who heard my stories many times and gave me the spark to write a book. Next, to Bryan Oettel, the editor at The Lyons Press who had the vision to see that within my ponderous manuscript was a fine story to tell. To freelance editor Richard Marek, who stimulated me to express my deepest feelings. And especially, thank you to Becky Koh, my spirited editor at The Lyons Press who believed in the book and provided the guidance and enthusiasm to carry it through.

There is also the practical world of producing a book. I thank my beleaguered secretary, Ginger Mitchko, for her uncanny ability to manage office crises during my frequent absences while at the same time providing me with unswerving loyalty and encouragement. Thank you also to my typists, Marilyn D'Aleo and Rochell Garmise, who, each time they were unreasonably asked to have the manuscript finished "yesterday," somehow were able to do it. And to my summer secretary in France, Marylène Bouchard, "un grand merci!"

I am deeply indebted to all the climbers with whom I've shared the mountains—for their high-spirited companionship but even more, for their long conversations, quiet reflections, and random comments. They have offered me a wealth of wisdom, insights, and humor, the best of which I hope has found its way into this book.

I've always depended on the support of my family and they've always come through: My brother Jerry Kamler and his wife, Marilyn, who are with me in spirit on all my adventures; my brother-in-law Jean-Paul Courchia, a fellow doctor and artist, and his wife Muriel, for their enthusiasm and encouragement; my in-laws, Louisette and Jacques Courchia, for all their kindness without being asked; my parents, Ethel and Willie Kamler, for their unlimited love and devotion; Burro who, besides correcting my English all through school, filled my world with optimism and positive thinking; and Potoff who, though he never climbed a mountain, showed me, before he left this world, what real courage was.

Like all my expeditions, writing this book required enormous support and sacrifice from the innermost ring of my shelter—the three people who enclose the happy place in which I live: Jonathan and Jennifer, who share with me their world of endless wonders and delights; and Josiane, who loves and understands me like no one else—my copilot and secret weapon. Nothing is impossible if I see my reflection in her bright eyes.

INTRODUCTION

Imagine a place so unnatural that the animals living there are barely aware of the change of seasons. Cold, wind, rain, and darkness, once controlling natural elements, have largely been reduced to periodic inconveniences. Absolute rules of nature have been comfortably disconnected, and a comprehensive artificial construction has replaced most of the natural landscape.

The sun rose over a parking lot outside my office at the lowest spot on the horizon between the hospital and the administration building. The beams aimed at my face, originating millions of miles away, were intercepted in the last tiny fraction of their journey by a tinted pane of glass. Their heat and light were effectively neutralized by air-conditioning and overhead lighting, but I knew it was morning because the sun was projected on my window. Though I couldn't feel it, there were indirect signs that it was a warm, breezy day: The guard was telling a patient in a top-down convertible he couldn't park here and short skirts were rustling as nurses came in to work. I was watching a silent movie from behind my desk.

Thinking about the day ahead had already made me tired. I had come in early to clear up the massive pile of papers on my desk but so far I'd done a lot more staring out the window. Soon my first patients would arrive and I'd have to start acting like a doctor: putting my tie on, being confident and sociable, and never making a mistake in any of my forty or so performances of the day. By the time I finished I'd be too worn out to do the paperwork so I'd leave it for tomorrow, just like I did yesterday. But maybe today if there weren't any emergencies, I would find an excuse to be outside for a while. . . .

"Did you take care of those notes on your desk yet?" my secretary, Ginger, said as she opened the door and walked in. Her matter-of-fact voice told me she knew beyond a doubt I hadn't. My rambling thoughts and imagination rapidly evaporated. Back to my ecological niche.

"Mrs. Chenkin called again today and says she is still in excruciating pain and why didn't you call her back last night?"

"I did. She wasn't home."

"I know. She said she was out bowling but she wants you to call her again this morning. Mr. Courchia called. He said you told him to soak his hand in warm water three times a day but yesterday he soaked it four times by mistake and now he doesn't know what to do about it."

"Couldn't you handle that?"

"I tried. I told him it was okay but he wants to hear it from the doctor. And when are you going to answer that letter that's been on your desk for two weeks?"

"Which one?"

"The one from the Hospital Utilization Review Office that wants to know why you delayed surgery a day on that guy who caught his hand in the clothes dryer. Their records show a 'so-called emergency' being admitted on the twenty-second, and yet surgery wasn't done until the twenty-third. The insurance company is refusing payment for the excess hospital day."

"I tried to explain to them on the phone that the patient was admitted to the E.R. at eleven-thirty at night and we started surgery at two A.M.—that's two and a half hours later. What more do they want?"

"They want it in writing. Then you have to call Mrs. Krantz. Her bandage is dirty and . . ."

"Could you bring me a cup of coffee?"

"Sure."

Drinking coffee with my feet up on the desk and looking out the window is one of the true simple pleasures of life. The sun was a little higher now, the trees and grass in the parking lot were greener, and there were more people walking around.

The view outside was better than the view inside. My walls are too bare, but I'm afraid if I fix up the office it will enclose me. Long years of studying followed by confinement to the hospital for 120 hours a week during my residency left me apprehensive, almost resentful, that life was passing me by. My profession was beginning to seem like a life sentence.

At unexpected moments, my work reminds me how ephemeral life is. It can pass quickly, like it did on the night I cut away a tuxedo from a man who had been hit by a car. His wife, semihysterical outside, was wearing an elegant red evening gown. The husband's cuff links matched the wife's necklace. I couldn't help thinking how much care they must have given to that detail a few hours earlier and how ridiculously trivial it seemed now.

Life is temporary even when it passes as slowly as an old lady who brought a muffin to her unresponsive, comatose husband every morning. "It's your favorite kind, blueberry," she said to him, pretending he could hear. How she must have wished that he would take that muffin and eat it, just like he used to—an act she probably always took for granted. She sat with him, fixed his hair, and at the end of visiting hours, wrapped the muffin back up and took it home.

At one time, I was desperately afraid of growing old without appreciating life while I was still able. Too soon, it seemed, the little boy in me was fading away as I accelerated along the prescribed route to become a member of the medical establishment. In my last year of residency, a respected elderly surgeon remarked that if business didn't pick up soon, he wouldn't be able to pay his maid. Then he asked me if I wanted to join his practice. It would be easy to slip into the lifestyle where success means staying ahead of your bills. Money certainly makes life easier but it's an add-on, not a substitute. I knew that, looking back, I'd regret what I didn't do far more than what I didn't own. Money wouldn't be a good answer if I wondered, too late, where my life had gone.

I had already sacrificed a large portion of it to become a doctor—an undertaking which gave me predictable rewards but also a serendipitous one. I went to medical school in southern France. One sunny day a girl called me up because she heard there was an American around and she wanted to practice her English. Josiane was cute, smart, sensitive, and strong—a rare combination, so I married her.

I relied on her strength during my residency, a demanding time over which I felt I had very little control. I was looking forward to my allotted vacation in my fourth year, but shortly before it was to start Josiane's father got sick and she flew off to France to help him recover—another reminder, a gentle one this time, of how people's lives can change in an instant. Suddenly, I had two weeks off with no idea what to do. But I did have an idea. There is nothing as real as a dream, and if you hold on to it it will always be there no matter what else changes. In my mind, I climbed back up the shelf and dusted off that old book.

After so many years of thinking it was inaccessible, I made a bridge from one world to another with a phone call—to a climbing school in New Hampshire. My instructor was an ex–Green Beret from North Dakota with whom it seemed I had nothing in common, but I loved climbing and we hit it off immediately. He turned out to be a sensitive soul with a spirit of adventure, something I felt I was too, but like drops of water from the same lake that flow into different rivers, we had traveled different paths and had mountains between us.

Six months later he asked me if I wanted to go climbing in Peru. This was my chance to be a real mountaineer, just like in the book. Josiane would have preferred that I stay home but she recognized that it was a chance to go down the road not taken. It would make me a more fulfilled person and she didn't want anything less for a husband, so she became my most enthusiastic supporter.

The hospital wouldn't like it. I'd have to flim-flam the schedule to take a month off, but I was chief resident, so I could do it and be gone before they noticed. Whatever happened afterward, I would have had my chance to climb.

"They might fire me, you know."

"Lifestyle is more important than resumé," Josiane said firmly. "You'll still find a job."

I went to Peru, climbed some mountains, and even became a local hero when I took care of a load of villagers and animals after their open truck overturned and rolled down a ravine in a remote area. I came back to New York having lived an adventure I had always dreamed about.

The doctors in the hospital seemed to admire what I had done, and (maybe not surprisingly) the elderly surgeon most of all. Only a token punishment was imposed but even had it been more severe, it would have been worth it. I had breathed some fresh air and regained my perspective. I returned enthusiastic for climbing, for medicine, for Josiane, and for everything else. I had made the right choice.

* * *

Ginger buzzed me on the intercom.

"The emergency room is on line one—something about a chopped hand."

Apparently it was still hanging, but just barely, from the arm of a nineteen-year-old female who decided to wear a gold bracelet this morning. Some guy tried to remove it with a hatchet.

I finished my coffee hoping there was more left in the cup than there was. This would be my last quiet moment for the rest of the day. I checked twice to be sure the cup was empty, then called Ginger back in.

"There's a near-complete amputation in the E.R. You'll have to cancel my schedule."

"I knew it. You always do this on our busiest days! Where do you want me to put everybody?"

"I don't know. Handle it."

"You have the easy part. Now I have to deal with all your patients. Don't forget to take your glasses and your microinstruments."

My office is two tree-lined parking lots away from the hospital, and the walk was my chance to be outside. It was, in fact, a warm breezy day but this would be the last I'd see of it.

Surgery is always an exhilarating and humbling experience. The human body is the most sacred of places, never meant to be entered, and accessible now only because of man's accumulated ingenuity. I'm grateful that some combination of forces in my life has granted me the privilege to cross the threshold into a fantastic realm few people will ever see.

In the operating room, the patient's hand, still dangling from the end of her arm, was placed on a table—a sort of workbench around which I sit with two surgery residents. A scrub nurse was within arm's reach, ready to pass me any instrument from her "tool bench." I was relieved to see I had an experienced team. As I have the reputation of being easy-going and never losing my temper, I often get paired with brand-new scrub nurses just out of school because I'm not likely to throw an instrument across the room no matter what is handed to me.

The hand is not some abstract organ like the liver or kidney. It's something with which we identify. Probably the only part of the body we take more personally is the face, so it's always hard to look at a mutilation. This one had a wedge-shaped gap at the end of the arm through which protruded a jumble of cut and dangling ropy-looking structures. The patient had what we call a "spaghetti wrist."

The first step was to bring order out of chaos. The microscope was lowered from the ceiling, and all the articulated arms were adjusted and tightened. Magnification and focus are controlled by foot pedals, so I took one sneaker off to have a finer touch with my toe. Nerves and tendons are both white, and with the blood long since drained from the hand, arteries and veins also appeared white. Laboriously we identified each structure and tagged it with a suture so we wouldn't lose it again. The hand is a superbly designed machine, but it would be a lot easier to fix if the parts were color-coded.

Once the inventory was complete, we began the repairs. Using needle-tipped forceps and a spring-loaded scissors with a tiny blade, I cut away all the damaged tissue edges. Then, with a suture so fine it's invisible without magnification, I began sewing. The needle, smaller than an eyelash, is held in a clamp and controlled by the tips of my thumb and index finger combined with a slight motion from the wrist. Tension on the knot has to be set by eye since the pull on the suture is too light to feel.

Strange as it sounds, the microrepairs were the least stressful part of the case. Spending hours working with my hands in deep concentration is profoundly relaxing and satisfying. The stress in a surgeon's life doesn't come from hard cases; meeting tough challenges that are sharply in focus is energizing. Stress comes from expending one's strength in poorly defined problems which may have questionable value and over which you have limited control. In surgery, the problem is clear, the goal is noble, and everyone in the room is doing his or her utmost to help you accomplish it. Besides, where else can you have people take you seriously while you are wearing pajamas, white socks, and tennis sneakers?

The ghostly hand suddenly turned pink as it was rejuvenated with fresh blood. With circulation restored, the time constraint for completing repairs was removed. The rest of the case would be easy.

"Dr. Kamler, there's a message from your wife. She wants to know if she should bring you dinner."

Jokingly I asked the residents, "Do you think you guys can get anything done while I'm scrubbed out?"

"We'll make better progress once you do" was the irreverent reply.

"Okay, tell her to come right away," I told the nurse.

I had been too preoccupied to think about eating or about Josiane, but realizing now that she had been aware of the emergency and was waiting to take care of me suddenly made me feel like we had been connected the whole day. I could have waited to eat until I got home, but I wanted her to understand how important that connection was for me. Sacrifices serve no purpose if we don't derive strength from them.

"I made you tuna patties and a potato omelette. And there is a big salad with my dressing that you like. Eat the tuna and omelette first while they're still hot. I guess you haven't eaten all day."

I was having a picnic supper on the coffee table in the O.R. lounge. My kids had come too. They never lose a chance to see "Daddy at work," and their faces were alive with excitement. Homework could wait.

Josiane opened a plastic container that was wrapped in a towel to keep it warm, and I started eating.

"See if it needs more salt. I brought extra salt in case you want. How is the case going?"

"Pretty good. The hand is pink again. We'll be finished in a few hours. It needs more salt."

My two children cavorted on one of the couches while several scattered doctors and nurses, eating pizza out of a cardboard box, looked on with amusement. Jonathan, who was eight years old, told me he definitely wanted to be a doctor when he grows up. Jennifer, who just turned six, was sure she wanted to wear a white coat, but was still undecided between doctor and ice cream man. I finished my salad and kissed Josiane good-bye. This happy little interlude was the perfect counterpoint to the intensity of the operating room.

A few hours later the patient was in the recovery room where the nurses were doting on her and checking the circulation in her fingers.

"Dr. Kamler, do you think the color of the fingers is okay?" one of the nurses asked, meaning she thought it wasn't.

I moved up to take a closer look. It wasn't. The fingers were mottled blue. If the vessels clotted off, I'd have to open her up and redo the repair. My heart sank as I contemplated the idea of going back to the O.R. instead of going home. I was hoping it was just a tight bandage and, several long seconds after loosening it, the finger color improved dramatically. I would be going home after all.

* * *

There is always a pot of coffee kept warm in the recovery room and there is always a sign above it that says "For Recovery Room Staff Only . . . Doctors This Means You." I took a cup anyway and walked out into the quiet, dimly lit lounge where there were two messages waiting for me. I sat down in the corner in an upholstered chair and cleared away the empty pizza box from the table in front of me so I could put my feet up. The first message was from a patient having surgery next week. He was at his girlfriend's house tonight and wanted me to call him there to discuss how soon after surgery they'd be able to go away on vacation. The second note was a reminder to do my charts before I left. I crumpled them both together and tossed them in the empty pizza box.

The next morning in my office, I sat down to a new pile of incomplete charts which had been placed on top of a previous pile of incomplete charts. Ginger came in with a stack of phone messages and an explanation of the new insurance coding procedures for surgery. I idly thumbed through my phone messages.

". . . so you have to use Code 6308 because 6307 has been deleted, unless you are not the primary surgeon, in which case—"

"Hey what's this message from Todd Burleson?"

"Oh, he said something about you and him going off to climb some mountain . . . I don't want to hear about it."

Ginger dreaded phone calls about mountains because they seemed inevitably to lead to long absences from the office. My climbing hadn't stopped after my residency despite Josiane's hope that it was just a phase I was going through. Climbing became my antidote for the stultifying effects of private practice, and I took regular doses in South America, Europe, and Antarctica. Todd's call however, was not about another "routine" climb. It was about Mount Everest. I already had a lot of experience climbing big mountains but this call could be my first chance to climb a legend.

As Ginger droned on, I reached over and dialed the phone. She stopped midsentence, but I assured her I was still listening to whatever it was she was talking about and she continued:

". . . but for any procedures entered with a BR rating, you have to submit a duplicate operative report unless—"

"Hello, Todd, I'm returning your call about climbing 'some mountain.' . . ."

Mount Everest has become the symbol for any supremely difficult goal that is almost, but not quite, out of reach. It's the ultimate challenge in any field of endeavor which, once undertaken, fires the spirit and drives the mind and body beyond their presumed limitations. I always assumed my challenge could never be the real Mount Everest. For me it would be sewing together blood vessels in mangled hands—certainly a worthy challenge but quite the opposite of climbing the world's tallest mountain. I was a surgeon. The powerful aura of Mount Everest had been absorbed by my subconscious and I considered its summit unattainable for me, though I had bypassed any conscious analysis of why that was so. But surgery was what I did, not what I was. Gradually I felt the need for a long pause from what I did in order to see what I was and whether there was any difference between the two.

People who climb big mountains actually live in a small world. I had never been to Asia but on whichever continent I climbed, I'd meet the same people and listen to the same stories, many of them first person accounts of attempts on Everest. Like any other mountain, or any goal in life, it was climbed one step at a time. After years of listening, I finally began to hear. I realized there was no one part I couldn't do if I didn't let the enormity of the challenge overwhelm me. Climbing Everest wasn't impossible. I was held back from trying by self-imposed limitations. The biggest barriers were in my mind.

Just the thought that I could climb Everest suffused me with an enthusiasm that shortened my sleep. I felt intensely alive and ready to tackle the Mount Everest of problems that I would have to solve before I could even get to Mount Everest.

I was a forty-four-year-old surgeon with a busy solo practice, devoted to my family and very married—enough strings to explain why I couldn't go off on a risky three-month expedition to the Himalayas. Thinking "I can't go" would settle me back into my familiar reassuring confinement. It would protect my self-image and prevent any future regret. *Can't* is often used when *won't* would be the more accurate word since it allows the user to feel the decision is out of his control. Sometimes fate leaves him no choice, but for me, for this goal, I knew that "can't go" really meant "won't go." Hard choices would have to be made and at some point in the planning I might decide to back off, but my present situation was determined by my previous choices and I wasn't ready to accept that I had no choices left. You don't close your options when you get old, you get old when you close your options. You can be old at any age. Climbing Everest would be the culmination of a boyhood dream and I still wanted to believe my horizon was limitless.

All my climbs start and end at home. For my trip to begin, Josiane had to believe in the idea. Everest would be longer and more dangerous than anything I'd ever done. Just extracting myself from my surroundings, let alone climbing the mountain, posed risks that she'd have to share. Once more I needed her enthusiastic support.

"The hardest part will be not having any contact with you for three months. I won't know what you're doing, how you're eating, whether you're sick or not. I won't even know when are the parts I should be worrying about."

"What good does it do to know when to worry?"

"What if you're doing something dangerous? I may not be thinking about you and you'll be alone."

After years of living with Josiane, these conversations actually made sense to me. Her thoughts, expressed with almost childlike innocence, reflected an unerring feel for the emotional currents that ran through our lives. With the family under constant bombardment from outside events, she maintains for us an island of quiet simplicity. I depend on it at home, in the operating room, and in the mountains.

Josiane finds her refuge in the family. She's scared of heights and big dogs, but she has the courage to follow her heart when it's for something she believes in. Though she is a doctor too, she put her career on long-term hold, enduring many disapproving glances from her colleagues, because she didn't want anyone else raising our children. Whenever she's asked her occupation, she replies "mother," not "doctor."

My refuge is in the mountains. As with surgery, I'm drawn there by the joy of concentrating all my energies—physical, mental, and spiritual—on one tangible goal. Survival on big mountains compels a focus so sharp that outside thoughts are forced into irrelevancy. Living so close to nature is intensely relaxing—rejuvenating. Josiane wishes I would find another way to relax but she empathizes with my feelings. She speaks of my climbing adventures with such animation and detail that listeners always assume she was there with me—and in a real sense, she was.

Spiritual considerations were nice to dwell on but practical problems intruded: "We won't have any income for a long time. What if the practice collapses while I'm gone? Doctors will find other surgeons to refer to. They'll forget who I am. Plus, when they find out what I'm doing, they'll think I'm an oddball."

"We always said we're not going to live our lives by what other people think and you're not going to be a prisoner of your practice. We don't owe any money. If the practice collapses, it collapses. You'll still be a doctor . . . and you'll still be an oddball, and I'll still be proud of you."

She was right: We always believed possessions own us more than we own them so we lived modestly, preferring to spend time rather than money. We lost out on acquisitions but we gained a lot in freedom.

Once we committed ourselves, pieces started falling into place. We could have called it luck but we prefer to believe that if you work hard to make something happen, your efforts will somehow be rewarded. Even if there seems to be no direct relation, there is a cosmic connection.

A permit to climb Everest is a precious commodity. In 1992, Nepal was granting only about one per year to any given country. They were very expensive, there was a ten-year waiting list, and even then, obtaining a permit depended on one's connections with the Nepalese government. At first it seemed I would have to wait a decade for a dubious outcome, but a climbing friend gave me the phone number of someone who was organizing a trip to Everest the following year. Todd Burleson ran a mountaineering school in Seattle called Alpine Ascents, and he was putting together a well-funded expedition sponsored in part by *National Geographic* for the purpose of mapping and measuring the exact height of Everest. Todd was picking climbers mostly from the West Coast, all of whom he had already climbed with. Besides not knowing me, my climbing resumé was a little thin by his standards. He said he'd get back to me. The return call to my office that day was to offer me a spot on the team. There were surely more-qualified climbers around, but he took me on as a sort of affirmative action program because he was anxious to have a doctor along.

I needed a place to train, but there aren't too many tall mountains in New York City. I cut back my work schedule so I could take frequent trips to New Hampshire to tune up and improve my climbing skills in the White Mountains. I joined a local YMCA near my office and finished off every workday with a one-mile swim to increase my overall fitness. My biggest need was to build endurance. There may not be mountains in New York City but there are skyscrapers. I used to live in a forty-story building on the east side of Manhattan that was so big the doorman didn't know that I moved out two years ago. I prevailed upon him to let me in at 5:00 A.M. and every day I drove there from my house in Queens. I climbed up the forty flights to the top, took the elevator down, and repeated it ten times. Four hundred flights and one-and-a-half hours later, I'd drive home across the Fifty-ninth Street Bridge before the morning rush hour traffic, take a shower and go to work.

My training was like a second job, but I took care to disturb family life as little as possible by taking the time out of my work schedule. My practice got more frenetic than ever as I tried to squeeze patients into less and less time.

The practice was thriving. I was willing to accept the collapse of the practice if need be, but I didn't want it to collapse. I had searched in vain for a temporary replacement. Hand microsurgeons are few and far between, and even rarer is one who has got nothing to do for three months. I was resigned to farming out my patients to other surgeons—something they were all too happy to help me with, given the competitive area in which I practiced.

As I was deciding which patients to send where, a pair of local surgeons split up. The divorce rate between doctors is probably higher than between doctors and their spouses. The junior partner was suddenly a doctor without a practice. I had a practice without a doctor. A perfect match. He could move into my office and keep my practice warm. When I explained the arrangement to my patients, they were delighted. Had I told them I was going off to play golf for three months, I'm sure the reaction would have been different but when they found out what I was doing they were very cooperative and supportive. Each wanted to "do his part" to help me along.

As Everest loomed larger, my family stood out in ever more vivid relief. I was painfully aware that my grand adventure would be harder on them than on me. I would be the one in a new and exciting environment. They would remain in familiar surroundings, feeling the hole created by my absence. A long pause in our daily rhythm might not be a bad thing, I told myself. It could serve as a contrast that would add vibrancy to our relationship when contact resumed. But what if it was more than a pause? There's an undeniable risk in climbing, and it's greater for those who stay at home. They had a lot invested in me. If I died on the mountain, they would suffer much deeper and longer than I would. My risk was undertaken voluntarily, but theirs was being imposed.

To justify going, I had to believe I could control the risk and that some risk was acceptable. More than once, I had backed off a climb when danger prevailed because of questionable weather or the need for skills beyond my level. I wasn't afraid to admit I was afraid and was proud of the reasoning and discipline I had shown in some of my failures.

Danger in the mountains is a reason not to climb, but it's also a reason to climb. It's not thrill seeking. Accepting risk means you gain immediate direct control of your life. It forces open your senses and puts your mind into sharp focus. You become a keen observer of nature's grand design and quiet nuances—the sights and sounds on which your survival depends. Thoughts and actions take on real-time intensity that's rarely achieved off the mountain. Risk is essential to the spirit of climbing. It's what elevates it above sport.

In the warm confines of home and family, the danger of climbing doesn't generate any fear at all. Abstract risk of death on a remote mountain is easier to accept than the very real deaths that surrounded me in the hospital; most of them due to natural biological causes but many due to "natural" societal causes like crime, accidents, drugs, pollution—the unavoidable risks of living in a spatially and spiritually compressed environment. True, the rewards of escape in the mountains carry their own set of risks, but I believed I could maintain a safe balance. Having treated a lot of climbers, I knew well enough that the dangers were real, and though stories of climbers' deaths abounded, so far I hadn't seen any up close. To climb Everest, I would have to raise the level of risk I found acceptable but I was a cautious climber, reassured by the reasoned belief that I could minimize the danger and also by the unreasoned belief that it wouldn't happen to me. I hadn't lost any friends to climbing—not yet. I left for Everest still enraptured by the poetry of the mountains.

CHAPTER

1

The first 11,415 miles are easy. TWA Flight 603 left JFK Airport, New York, at 4:30 P.M., March 21, 1992, with stops in Seattle, Washington; Tokyo, Japan; Bangkok, Thailand; Kathmandu, Nepal. In some areas, man has such mastery over nature that all it takes to go halfway around the world is an airplane ticket—economy class, no less. The ticket runs out after two days of flying. I'd step off the airplane into trekking shoes and take ten days to hike the next thirty miles along the trail. Only the last part of the journey would be hard. With nature firmly back in control, I'd switch to climbing boots and need about two months to try to go the last five miles up Everest.

Jonathan understood that it was "a big mountain" and that I'd be away "a long time," so I was a little puzzled by his rather casual good-bye at the airport. Jennifer sighed with relief when we reached the boarding gate and she realized that it was just me, not the whole family, who was going to climb Everest. Josiane was upset but preferred not to think about the big picture, instead transferring her anxiety to the apple she forgot to pack in my food bag. She did remember, though, to give me a note, to be read only after I was on the plane.

The flight across the Pacific outlasted five full-length movies, none of which I felt like watching. Several rows in front of me was a small, high-spirited group that I realized early on was part of my expedition. Being the only team member who hadn't climbed with any of the others, I was still anonymous, and wanted to remain that way a little while longer. There would be plenty of time to get to know each other. My thoughts were still at home and I needed to make the transition slowly. When the flight attendant brought around fruit, I was quick to take an apple so I could pretend it was the one Josiane forgot to give me. It seemed like a good time to unfold her note:

"Be careful. Remember how much you have waiting for you at home."

At our layover in Bangkok, I introduced myself to the group that had collected so far. Everyone was glad, and relieved, to meet the doctor. They were afraid I had missed the flight. The minigroup was led by Skip Horner—a professional river-runner and mountain guide from Montana. He had climbed extensively in the Himalayas but had never been to Everest. Adventure was nothing new to him. Hugh Morton was a banker from Atlanta. He had been training for Everest for years, but his job never allowed him the time to go. When the savings and loan scandal broke, he became unemployed. He believed his layoff was an act of God to give him a chance to climb. Perry Salmonson was a pilot for a small northwestern airline. He was young and, dressed in a tight tee-shirt, appeared to be the fittest of the group. The youngest was John Helenick. He was making a good living from his father's tool and dye business but anxious to accomplish something on his own. There was one woman—Margo

Chisholm. She was squarely built and strong and had climbed all over the world, but with her dangling earrings and gregarious personality, she reminded me of a suburban housewife from Connecticut (which was where she was originally from). We all sat around the hotel lobby discussing whether it was time to go to sleep or have breakfast.

At the end of our second day of flying, I was slowly beginning to hope the plane would crash, just to relieve the monotony, when the pilot announced we were entering Nepal and that Everest was visible out the window. Outside was a uniform carpet of clouds pierced by a single, massive triangle of black rock. Cruising at 29,000 feet, I was at eye level with the summit—impossibly remote, fearsome, and cold. What conceit to think any human could, or should, stand there.

The austere, majestic image was quickly erased as the plane descended below the clouds and I was pitched into the chaos of Kathmandu. The streets were overcrowded with noise, filth, cows, and people.

Nepal is a hybrid country. I saw it in the streets. Indian faces and Hindu culture have come up from the south; Tibetan faces and Buddhist culture have come down from the north. Sprinkled into the mix are Caucasian faces, some of which belonged to our expedition as we scurried about for a few days buying last-minute supplies; filling out forms and paying fees for visas, visa extensions, trekking permits, and climbing permits; submitting photos; and then submitting still more photos.

Our advance team had already been in Nepal for two weeks. Todd, the expedition leader, was at base camp. Pete Athans, our climbing leader, was still in town shuttling between various government bureaucracies trying to obtain clearances for the sophisticated and strange devices we needed to bring through customs: laser telescopes and reflectors, as well as global positioning satellite (GPS) beacons and recorders. It requires tons of equipment to measure centimeters on a mountain, but we hoped to come away with the most precise measurement ever of the height of Everest.

At the last minute, the Nepalese authorities balked at the idea: If a new altitude was to be determined, the information should come from Nepalese, not American, geologists. Worse, Everest is the only mountain over 29,000 feet. What if our measurements put the altitude below that rarefied level? And far worse, even calamitous, what if the measurements showed that Everest wasn't the world's tallest mountain?

Finding a way through the bramble of national pride and massive paperwork in which our equipment was snagged depended on Pete's diplomatic skills. He was a professional mountain guide from Colorado who had already summitted Everest twice. He spoke fluent Nepali, but even more important, he was soft-spoken and had endless patience.

My responsibility was our medical supplies, which included heavy doses of narcotics. I was requested to come to the customs house to clear everything personally. The inspector looked at the four captive trunks I'd packed strategically back in New York and randomly picked one for me to open. He rummaged inside and lifted out a twelve-pack of preloaded syringes filled with morphine. As I was calculating my probable jail time, he put it back, said "It's okay," and waved me through.

The only other medical item I needed to obtain was a supply of tinnabar—a drug that's illegal in the United States. It's a potent antibiotic that the FDA won't approve because it can cause a severe rash and there are other, tamer, antibiotics that work just as well against American germs.

Climbers have told me, however, that in Nepal they've occasionally been afflicted with a nearly unstoppable diarrhea that responds only to tinnabar. I had no trouble getting it at a local pharmacy—no prescription needed.

The pharmacy was one of many ancient brick buildings which lined narrow smoke-filled streets choked with cars and trucks that blew out black clouds of diesel exhaust. A policeman wearing a gas mask was directing traffic around a cow eating garbage in the road. The noise of a barking dog drew my attention to a butcher shop: a row of metal pails placed on the sidewalk in the hot afternoon sun, each filled with an assortment of animal parts. A dog had crept up to one pail and was pulling out a large piece of meat. A woman customer approached and grabbed the piece from the other side. A brief tug-of-war ensued until the dog was scared off. The woman put the meat back and then bought the whole pail.

Having done all my "medical stuff," I was free to take care of some personal errands—like getting a haircut, something I didn't have time to do before I left the States, and purchasing a pair of extralong laces for my hiking boots. Once everything on my list was crossed off, I still had some time left to be a tourist. I hailed a bicycle-powered rickshaw and took a ride up a hillside to the Swayambunath Temple—the holiest site in Kathmandu.

Riding up the hill, I intruded on homes without walls. Families were living on the sidewalk. With their household belongings carefully arranged around them, they were cooking meals on little burners and serving on plates placed directly on the cement ground. They carried on their intimate daily routines oblivious to casual observers like me.

The rickshaw crossed several bridges and some open fields. There were boys playing cricket and girls filling brass urns with water from stone wells. Women were doing their laundry in stagnant green water while their children bathed nearby. I wondered how dirty something or someone had to be to get cleaner with that water.

The temple was a large white dome on a terrace overlooking the valley. Monkeys inhabit every part of it and patrol the grounds looking for food. I didn't find it very inspiring, but the legend about it is:

A Tibetan god, Manjushri, came to see a lotus that was floating on a huge lake in Kathmandu Valley. The lotus was too far away for him to see, so with his sword he cut into the lake and drained it. The lotus came to rest at this spot on the mountain and so it was here the temple was built. The strange part is Kathmandu Valley actually was formed from a drained lake, but that discovery was made only recently.

On the return ride, my driver asked me how I liked Nepal. I said, "I thought there were supposed to be mountains around here but so far I haven't seen any."

He said, "A few years ago, the valley was clear and we could see mountains all around. As far as I know, they're still here."

Tomorrow I'd find out for sure when we flew into the foothills. It had taken three days for everyone, except Pete, to get their jobs done—a lot more time than I would have liked given that each meal here ran the risk of becoming a stomach adventure and each breath of air added another layer of black to our lungs—lungs that would soon be pushed to the limit in thin air. I was anxious to get everyone out of Kathmandu. Civilization has heavily affected this once-delicate city nestled in a high Himalayan valley.

Only Pete was staying behind, still frustrated in his attempt to untangle our key equipment. He said, "Either I'll catch up with you in a few days, or you'll hear on the radio that the interior minister has been murdered."

Back in my hotel room on the eve of our departure, I took a hot bath, removing the coating of Kathmandu from my skin and extracting one last bit of luxury before we dropped out of civilization. Too soon there was a knock on the door. Skip came in with a fish scale to weigh my bags for the plane ride tomorrow. Each one checked out okay. I was packed and I was clean. Physically, I was prepared to leave, but mentally, not quite yet. I had to make a phone call.

There's a thirteen-hour-and-fifteen-minute time change to New York. (Thirteen time zones I can understand, but why Nepal chooses to add an additional fifteen minutes is a mystery.) Evening calls here become early morning calls there, but Josiane answered on the first ring. Anticipating I might call, the whole family had fallen asleep on the couch to be near the phone. It was sad to think I was so far away from them, and I had to remind myself I was doing this voluntarily.

Josiane explained the reason for Jonathan's casual good-bye at the airport. After coming home, Jonathan sat in front of the window and fell asleep trying to wait up for me. That was his idea of "a long time."

I had called Josiane at each step along the route, from the West Coast, Japan, Thailand, and now Nepal. She said she felt as if I was disappearing over the horizon. Tomorrow I would be over the edge and she wouldn't hear from me for the next two months.

"I'm going to worry about your plane ride tomorrow. After that I won't know what's going on, but remember I'll be thinking about you all the time. When you need strength, we'll still be connected."

At ten dollars a minute, I couldn't say all I suddenly felt. When I'm about to lose her is when I realize how much she means to me. Though her emotions ride close to the surface, mine are carried deeper down, usually covered by the temporary distractions of routine life that add up to a permanent layer that prevents me from expressing, or even realizing, what's there. It takes moments like these to bring them to the surface.

No matter how far away I go, Josiane keeps me centered. She likes the bold mountain man, cowboy-doctor image others have of me, but she also understands, like no one else could, that my motivation springs from a chronic anxiety that I haven't accomplished enough with my life, haven't reached my potential. Because she can admire my strengths while understanding my weaknesses, she sees me, and makes me see myself, as I truly am. She is the only one for whom I really need to be a hero.

That was what I was thinking. What I said was "I love you and I'll miss you," or something like that.

We hugged each other through the phone and I hung up still feeling like we were holding hands. The call was just what I needed. I could now turn my strength toward the mountain with equanimity and single-minded concentration.

CHAPTER

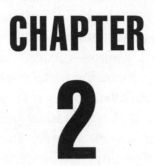

My Kathmandu alarm clock—a diesel truck—went off earlier than usual in the morning. I was awakened, not by the noise of the engine idling in the street, but by the diesel fumes leaking in around the window frame and choking me. I sought refuge in the bathroom only to find my roommate, Perry, already there on the floor doing sit-ups. My first thought was not to let myself get psyched out by the other climbers on this trip. A few extra sit-ups here and there were not going to make any difference and even more, if Perry felt like he needed to do sit-ups now, maybe he just lacked confidence. My second thought was, maybe I should be doing sit-ups too.

Our exit from civilization was the airport's Domestic Departure Terminal, a dilapidated brick building with a dirt floor and people and baggage everywhere. Among the crowd was another member of our expedition for me to meet: Frank Fischbeck—refined, reserved, and very British. A former *Time-Life* photographer, he lived in Hong Kong where he owned FormAsia, a small publishing company. He had been staying at a different hotel than the rest of us because he "preferred the accommodations there." Others in our group who had climbed with him vouched for Frank as a dependable team player, but he was quiet and slow to integrate himself into a group—qualities with which I easily identified. I liked Frank immediately. Besides, he was one of the few expedition members older than I.

There were two flights to Lukla, our destination, each capable of holding sixteen people, and there were three hundred waiting to get on: Nepalis anxious to go home and trekkers anxious to begin their adventure in the Himalayas. The besieged airport manager said, "Absolutely not," when we asked if there was any chance we could get on the plane. That was before he opened the envelope Pete had given us to give him if there was a problem. The rupees disappeared into his pocket, leaving only a piece of paper with the names of our expedition members on it. He carefully underlined each name and said, "Maybe."

If we were lucky all we would have to do was stand around and wait, but I wasn't so lucky. I suddenly had to go to the bathroom, and I mean suddenly. I found the bathroom just in time. There was one clogged toilet and people had obviously been using the floor and walls instead. In the corner I spotted two footrests with a hole in the floor between them. I accomplished my immediate goal, but I wasn't at all sure now about my larger goal of escaping Kathmandu without getting sick.

A few boring hours later we got called, one by one, into a closet-sized room called a Check Point. Security control turned out to be a guard who, once the curtain was closed around us, pointed to my knapsack and said, "You give money, I no look."

"Go ahead, look."

"It's okay," he said, and waved me through. On the other side, everyone said he did the same to them, and several people actually gave him money.

There were no reserved seats on the Twin Otter, but boarding was arranged so that the distribution between the light-weight Sherpas and us climbers, each at least sixty to seventy pounds heavier, would keep the plane balanced.

The door to the cockpit was open and the pilot joked with us that he tried to avoid flying through clouds because "Around here, clouds sometimes have mountains in them." As we came in for the landing I could see through the windshield, a dirt strip straight ahead of us cut into the slope, somewhat leveled but still decidedly uphill and ending abruptly at a cliff face. It didn't help my confidence any to see a crashed plane lying off to the side of the runway.

We landed safely and stepped out onto a dirt field. As the plane was unloaded, we separated our gear from the lumber, chickens, rolls of fabric, and other cargo. When the plane took off again, it occurred to me that that would probably be the last loud noise I would hear for the next two months. I wished there were some way to tell Josiane we landed safely (she worries about plane rides more than anything else) but I was now out of communication with the outside world. No transportation; no telephone; not even a beeper. Instead of being frightening, the idea was relaxing. I was definitively cut off from the routines and concerns of everyday life and free to immerse myself in the experience that was about to unfold.

"Over here, over here," called out a friendly Tibetan face.

We crossed the landing field to a crowd of Sherpas and yaks and I felt like I was walking back two centuries in time.

"Welcome to Lukla," said Ong-Chu, our official greeter. He was the expedition's base camp leader, charged with the logistics of getting all our supplies to base camp, then cooking our meals and generally running the place as smoothly as possible so we could concentrate on climbing.

A stream of Sherpas moved past me to tend to the gear. The landing field is the staging area for transshipment from plane to yak so that material can be transported into the remoter regions of the Himalayas.

A phalanx of yaks was led onto the field and waited patiently for their assignments. Sherpas uncoiled ropes and placed blankets and wooden frames on the backs of the yaks. My responsibility at each step was for the medical supplies, and I had to be certain that all the trunks made it this far still intact. Satisfied that they were, I gave the okay to Ong-Chu and he gave the order to some of his Sherpa crew to go ahead and load them.

Sitting on the floor of my office in New York surrounded by $30,000 worth of medical supplies and state-of-the-art equipment, I had given a great deal of thought to how it all should be packed. Fragile equipment like ophthalmoscopes had to be wrapped inside softer supplies like bandages. Heavier supplies like casting material and bags of IV fluids had to be distributed among all the containers to make the loads bearable. Supplies had to be separated so that if any one container was lost or crushed, it wouldn't be a critical loss to the expedition.

I had managed to pack everything into four heavy-duty plastic trunks. They were a lot heavier than I thought they'd be and I had images in my mind of dirty looks from angry Sherpas as they forced the loads onto yaks that staggered under the weight.

The loading began and I watched, with some trepidation, for the reaction from the Sherpas as they lifted the first medical trunk. There wasn't any. They continued their amiable conversation as they adjusted the load, and even the yak didn't seem to mind. As if to reassure me further, once they tied the trunk on, they added more bags on top—the trunk wasn't even a full load for the yak.

I watched the supply train pull out. The brightly colored trunks on sale in the basement of Sears one week ago were now a cultural aberration on the backs of yaks heading up a remote mountain trail in central Asia.

The sun was gone and it was getting cold. I reached into my knapsack to pull out another sweater. We were at eight thousand feet. The air was thin and didn't hold much heat. Once the sun is blocked by the mountains the cold returns quickly. My breathing was more rapid, but I thought it was due to the excitement.

We entered a teahouse with a sign outside on which was neatly printed, "Good Lodging and Fooding." The simple square room with wooden tables and benches was empty until the proprietor appeared and handed us menus. A misplaced comma made for an intriguing item: "If you sleep here and eat bed, 20 rupees." We agreed that twenty rupees was a pretty reasonable price to eat a bed but we decided to order more traditional food: boiled potatoes, fried bread, and Coca-Colas.

Soon, it was time to get going. Sherpas have lived at this altitude for five hundred years but we'd been here barely one afternoon. We had just come up six thousand feet in elevation and I was concerned about altitude sickness—a well-described but not well-understood condition that causes headaches and vomiting and can lead to life-threatening conditions if not controlled. As with any disease, the best way to treat it is to not get it in the first place. That means making as gradual an ascent as practical and, whenever possible, sleeping at a lower elevation than the maximum altitude for the day. This gives the body its best chance to adjust to the lower amount of oxygen in the air. Our planned sleeping point was Phakding, a village only a short hike away. At an altitude nine hundred feet lower than Lukla, it was the logical place to rest so our first night's breathing would be as easy as possible. The Chinese have categories for mountains, either "big headache" or "little headache." We were on our way to the ultimate "big headache mountain," and by going slowly, we'd get there faster.

Besides the medical reasons, as a climber I was also anxious to get going. Not "to get to the mountain already" as some of the team members professed, but to begin to test myself, to make sure that even if I wasn't fully up to the task of climbing Mount Everest, at least I wouldn't be an embarrassment to myself along the way. Probably some of the other first-timers on Everest felt the same way but no one said so.

Skip took the lead to show us the way. I told everyone it was prudent for the doctor to lag behind because if anyone broke down on the trail, I'd come upon him. The truth is, I like to be alone with my thoughts when I hike. A Sherpa was assigned to follow close behind me, carrying a fishing tackle box that I had prepared with medical supplies that might be needed along the way. My Sherpa "caddy" would also be looking out for me in case I was the one who broke down.

There are no roads here—just narrow trails that connect one village to another. There is no flat land—paths run up, down, and around the mountains and are far too steep and rocky for any wheeled vehicles. Transportation is entirely by foot power—human or yak. At this altitude the trail is hard-packed dirt, well worn and easy to follow. It starts up over the top of a slope and then descends gradually down the other side. I set off at a good pace and felt fit.

The trail descended to the river and Phakding was just ahead across a narrow wood-and-cable suspension bridge.

I came into town (two teahouses) feeling proud of myself but trying to look like this was all routine. Most of the other climbers and quite a few trekkers had already arrived and were drinking Cokes with their feet up. I took the outside stairs to the second floor and put my pack down on one of a row of wooden bunks to lay claim to a sleeping space that I would move into once my duffel bag arrived. It was still en route on the back of a yak or possibly the back of a Sherpa. To keep our backpacks light, we tried to carry just those things we might need during the day, like snacks, water, and extra clothes. My tee-shirt was soaked with sweat, and with the sun gone, I got cold as soon as I stopped moving. I stripped off the shirt, changed to the spare one in my pack, put the rest of my clothes back on minus a few layers, and went back down to the teahouse. Having come through my first day successfully, I was now more in the mood to socialize.

Fatigue and clean quiet air combined to give me a good night's sleep. The diesel truck that had awakened me yesterday already seemed long ago and far away. I was receding into a simpler time.

I arrived late for breakfast, but before anyone had a chance to mock me for it I announced that today was a day to take it slow and, "As your doctor, I'm setting a good example."

I started in on my omelette and fried bread.

"How'd you sleep?" I asked Mike Gordon in an offhand manner. Mike had joined up with our group en route yesterday. He was new to me but well known to many of the others. He was an experienced climber from Alaska, and this would be his second attempt on Everest. He had flown in a few days earlier to get a jump on his acclimatization, something that had given him a problem last year.

"I slept okay," Mike replied to my question, "except I think yesterday's boiled chicken gave me a nightmare."

"How about you, John?"

"Well, I would have slept well except I woke up every time Margo tried to unzip my sleeping bag."

"Yeah," said Mike, "that was my nightmare, too."

Amid the general laughter, I actually was making rounds, finding out as casually as I could, how each climber had slept and how much they were eating—important indicators as to how they were acclimatizing. Spirits seemed high but we were in a group now. I would have preferred to ask each climber in private but I had gotten up too late. Sometimes the answers are very different when you have the person alone.

The plan today was to go on up to Namché Bazaar, an elevation gain of three thousand feet. I wasn't looking for any hiking companions, so I tried not to start off at the same time as anyone else. Frank and I finished packing at about the same time but I sensed in him the same need for solitude that I had and we easily found reasons to not leave together.

Walking upstream along the Imja Kola River I felt part of it. The blue-green water smashing against the rocks sent up a sparkling mist that hung over the valley. It covered me with fine droplets of water, a welcome cooling for my sweaty, grimy skin after two hours of hiking in the sun. The trail ran along the scoured rock at the river's edge. It crossed the river several times over low wooden bridges that cleared the water by means of rock piles placed on either bank, upon which the bridge rested. When the waters flood, these bridges routinely wash out and have to be rebuilt. Alongside one of them was a neatly stacked pile of lumber ready to be made into the next bridge. I was absorbed by the noise and turbulence of this river, which takes its source from the flanks of Everest. What powerful gods there must be up ahead.

The countryside was beautiful, and surprisingly delicate for such a harsh environment. Juniper, pine, and rhododendron trees covered the hillsides and filled the air with a fragrant, ever-changing combination of scents. Scattered huts that we passed along the way were made of chiseled stones with corners cut perfectly square. The doors and windows were framed with brightly painted wood. Everyone we met said "Namasté" and very quickly we took to saying it in reply. It's the official all-purpose hello–goodbye Sherpa greeting.

The open space above the river got narrower as the hills closed in on both sides and the valley turned into a gorge. The path steepened into a series of switchbacks along one side, up to a cliff overlooking the turbulent river now far below and almost silent. The trail continued on the other side, the two parts linked together by a high-flying suspension bridge: two steel cables bolted to opposite sides of the gorge, with a narrow wooden trestle hanging in between. With no other anchoring points, the long bridge sagged in the middle and swayed rhythmically with the wind, all the more so if a yak happened to be crossing at the same time as you. The floorboards were rotted out at irregular intervals, the holes sometimes covered by planks dropped loosely over them, sometimes not. Crossing the bridge meant watching my feet every step of the way, with far too many scenic views between my legs of the river far below.

Getting to the other side of the bridge gave me the chance to do the same thing many more times on up the road. This land is riddled with incredibly steep, precipitous gorges cut by powerful rivers. The land has been uplifting for the last fifty million years, ever since the Indian plate collided with the Asian plate and started sliding under it, causing the Asian plate to wrinkle. The "wrinkles" are now the Himalayas—the highest mountains in the world. They are still rising. Just how rapidly was one of the measurements we were here to make.

A hot sun had been out most of the day but now, more and more, it was disappearing behind clouds or being blocked by high ridges. I didn't know whether to take off my tee-shirt or put on a sweater. Before I could decide, the trail wound around a final bend and Namché was before me.

Once a remote village tucked into a steep horseshoe-shaped valley, Namché has been prospering relentlessly as a weekly marketplace for hundreds of years and as a rest stop for climbers and trekkers for the last fifty. The population has grown to nine hundred. All the houses are rectangular, two stories high, made of stone but covered with clay and lime to block the wind. Windows and doors always face southeast to let in as much warming sun as possible. The houses are built on rings of terraced land that ascend the slopes on all three sides, each ring wider than the one below, giving the town the look of a football stadium.

This year there was a dispute over water rights. Villagers who live higher up laid pipes to divert a stream that flowed through the town, greatly distressing the inhabitants below. A local citizen coalition was formed, which resolved the issue, at least temporarily, by smashing the pipes with axes.

The remainder of today, and all day tomorrow would be time for rest. As a general rule, it's not a good idea to gain more than two thousand feet every three days. We were at our physiological limit and it was time to pause. If everyone was doing well tomorrow, we'd move up the following day. If not, we'd take an additional day here. If really not, we'd back down.

Tea was served by a little girl in traditional Sherpani dress. Through the window I watched a group of children

playing with a goat and beyond them, yaks uprooting potatoes in a dirt field. Between orders, the girl tended to her little brother, swathed in robes of various colors that had
faded generations ago. Her older sister wore tight dungarees
and a New York Mets tee-shirt.

The teahouse, being new, was on the uppermost ring of
the village. Far below, but not so far away was Ong-Chu's
house, visible and within shouting distance for the Sherpani
big sister who stood on top of a stone wall and called down
to him. He had invited our group for dinner and she wanted
to know if he was ready for us yet. He answered on the second yell, coming out of his house and motioning to her to
send us down. It was the Sherpa telephone.

The path wound its way between terraces and along
roofs, at times descending so steeply and narrowly that,
walking single-file and facing inward, the person ahead was
at eye level with the knees of the person next behind.

"Welcome," said Ong-Chu's wife, smiling as she placed
her fingertips together, pointing them under her chin and
nodding to each of us.

"Namasté," we replied, as we entered her house one by
one, ducking our heads to get through the low wooden door.

We were in the stable—the lower level where the animals
were kept in the winter when it was too cold for them to be
outside. There was a low ceiling, dirt floor, and raw stone
walls. Set off in one corner was a small alcove—a family
chapel with smooth walls, pictures, decorations, and statuary. A wooden ladder led us up through a hole in the ceiling
to the second floor—a large open area with a wooden floor
and a fireplace in the middle. The walls were lined with cup-
boards, and the shelves were filled with food containers,
canned goods, blankets, and pots and pans. This was the all-
purpose room for entertaining, conducting business, and
sleeping. The fire is the center of all Sherpa activities.

Ong-Chu greeted each of us upstairs with a handshake and a glass of *chang*—the local moonshine made from fermented barley and guaranteed to keep you warm on even the coldest of Himalayan nights. Many of our group partook despite my reservations. Alcohol and altitude don't mix, but what concerned me even more was that the water used to make it hadn't been boiled and therefore was certainly contaminated. My objections, however, were overruled by a lot of backslapping and a consensus that the alcohol content was so strong it would kill anything swimming in it.

Dinner was *momos*—meat wrapped in noodles—a dish that is served probably everywhere, but called wonton, ravioli or kreplach depending on the country. Ong-Chu's wife (we called her Mrs. Ong-Chu because we didn't know her first name and Sherpas have no last names) couldn't speak English but was the perfect hostess, attentive to each of us. The yak meat tasted awful, but to be polite I took some on my plate and made believe I was eating it. I thought I was doing a good job but I didn't fool her. Without commenting, she got up from the table and came back with a bowl of vegetable and rice soup that she placed before me.

The dinner was winding down. Mrs. Ong-Chu replaced the wood in the fireplace with dried yak dung. Wood is a relatively scarce commodity here but it's burned when a high temperature is needed for cooking. For warmth, burning yak dung is sufficient and more economical.

As we leaned back on our yak-skin-covered wicker stools and drank tea, Ong-Chu proudly showed us his collection of fine bronze, copper, and iron pots which took up several shelves along one wall. Besides being a measure of wealth among the Sherpas, it reflected the light from the fireplace and filled the room with a warm glow as night descended outside.

As we left, Mrs. Ong-Chu placed a prayer shawl around each of us. You could see the relief in her face. She had just had a dinner party and everything went well. Personality transcended nationality and no common language was needed to understand her emotions.

Rest day was market day. The market is over at about 8:00 A.M. so seeing it means getting up early. Easier for some of us than for others: "Man, my head hurts" was a comment I heard more than once.

"Hey, too much chang last night!" was the common rejoinder. Maybe, but maybe not. Too much altitude can have the same effect. A headache is often an early sign of altitude illness, and last night had been our first night at almost twelve thousand feet. A chang headache will clear up. An altitude headache will get worse. We'd take a leisurely stroll in the market and let time sort it out.

Leisurely was not the word for this market. It's held in the flattest spot in town: two switchbacks on the slope directly above Ong-Chu's house, and it's packed with people from all over the Khumbu region. Hindu-looking farmers from the lower valleys sit on the ground selling vegetables laid out on towels. Tibetan herders, who come through the mountain passes, stand next to animal carcasses hanging from the rock walls. They hold long knives, ready to cut up any part of the animal you wish to buy. Sherpa traders sell canned food from India and soap from China. The market was overflowing with noise and motion. Gradually I worked my way out. There was nothing for me to buy and I was afraid of stepping on somebody's vegetables, knocking a kid or a chicken off the cliff, or angering a Tibetan with a long knife.

Our group reassembled after the market and I was pleased to learn all headaches were gone, confirming the diagnosis of chang overdose. I encouraged everybody to go for a short hike to expose themselves briefly to higher altitude. Two climbers went up to a monastery on the ridge but no one else took my advice, not even me. My biggest exertion for the day was walking down the hill to the "post office"—the last one on the way to Everest. It was somebody's house, in front of which was a small garbage can bolted to the wall. The mailman got up from his potato field, brought me in his house, and gave me some stamps. Then he gestured for me to drop my mail in the garbage can on the wall outside, which I now realized was the mailbox. I reached in with my other hand first, reassured myself by feeling some other letters and then let my postcards drop.

At dinner I learned the hike to the monastery had been a fiasco. The trail was much longer than it looked. When the climbers finally arrived, they asked the monk for a blessing, but he refused, saying it was his day off.

The dinner was a special treat. Sliced goat meat served on a tray with the cooked head of the goat, eyes wide open, sitting upright in the center. Somehow none of us were very hungry. I might have made an attempt to eat a piece if I hadn't realized with a shock that the goat the children had been playing with yesterday wasn't around today.

It was time to leave Namché. Except for a few cases of diarrhea (which I felt obligated to ask about in greater detail than I really wanted to hear), everyone seemed to be healthy. No headaches, no bizarre behavior (which can also be a sign of altitude illness), except maybe for Frank. I knew he was fastidious, but this morning after he rolled up his sleeping bag, he wouldn't leave his bunk until he squared off the corners and tucked in the sides of the filthy blanket that the teahouse provided. He was making his bed. It was definitely time to leave Namché.

"Every time I take a breath, I'm glad to get something," a trekker said to no one in particular as he rested at the top of the hill leading out of Namché. I would have agreed with him except I didn't want to waste any breath talking. Starting out today, we were all feeling the thin air. All of us, that is, except the children of Namché who passed us in droves on their way to school. Every day they came up this trail and then turned off down to their school on the other side of the mountain. And some of them came home for lunch. It was too demoralizing to rest here. I continued on past the kids' turnoff so I could be alone and conjure up a more flattering image of myself unimpeded by reality.

Mercifully, the trail leveled off and then snaked around several grassy slopes, gradually descending toward the river. It was a broad path of hard-packed dirt and was easy going. The air was cool but the sun was out and it was a perfect day for a jaunty hike. The trail descended more steeply and again I was surrounded by tall trees and the roar of the river.

In the Himalayas, what comes down must go up. Our destination today was Thangboché, a monastery one thousand feet higher than Namché, but so far today I'd steadily descended. It wasn't hard to figure out what awaited me on the other side of the river, but there's only so many times you can adjust your pack, retie your shoes, and admire the view before you have to start off again.

Gongs sounded and cymbals clashed just as I arrived at the top of the plateau. The sound from the monastery was overwhelming, breaking the silence of two hours alone on a steep dusty trail. It was so perfectly timed with my arrival that I was sure it was for me. The scene was ethereal. Ahead of me on a broad open plain was the imposing Thangboché Monastery. Behind it was a backdrop of impossibly tall ice mountains so sharply outlined in the thin cold air that they must have been made of cardboard. There was a layer of clouds and then the mountains continued above them. The peaks of the tallest ones were obscured by a white blend of snow, ice, clouds, and mist.

Chomolungma, the goddess mother of the earth, as the Sherpas call Everest, was still veiled. We had entered her kingdom but she was not yet ready to make an appearance.

Our Sherpa support team had arrived well ahead of me and was efficiently setting up our tents on the expanse in front of the monastery. There were some teahouses on the other side of the field but the higher we went the smaller and less sanitary they became, and here it seemed about time to move into tents—colder but cleaner. I could have safely offered my help to the Sherpas because I was sure they wouldn't accept but I was too tired even to make a pretense. Finding a comfortable spot between two large stones, I sat down and watched as the Sherpas unloaded the yaks, letting them roam over the field with the looming monastery on the left, the ramshackle teahouses on the right, the over-powering mountains all around. It was a timeless scene, un-changed for five hundred years—except for one glaring anomaly: our half-dozen high-tech state-of-the-art dome tents brought here by beings from another world who were slowly co-opting the local population and subverting their culture.

Should I feel guilty about being one of the invaders? Technology has just now progressed to the point where it's possible to put regular humans, not just supermen, into the most extreme areas on earth. But the same technology ho-mogenizes those areas. They become easier to visit but, little by little, less worth visiting. Earlier access was denied be-cause of their remoteness. Future access will be denied be-cause they will have passed into history.

It was getting cold. The high plateau was exposed to the winds that swept down from the snowy slopes. I hadn't yet answered my own question but it was time to move. I got up and put on two jackets. The wind blew away some of the cloud cover and suddenly Everest came into view. The peak jutted up just above the surrounding mountains—a black triangle, in sharp contrast to the icy white peaks around it. Everest is so high it's in the jet stream, a current of wind that circles the earth at eighty miles an hour. The winds scour the peak and don't let snow accumulate, blowing it off into the sky in a long trailing plume clearly visible from where I stood, sixteen thousand feet below. The view was awesome. The point of that black triangle was the highest point on earth. Chomolungma.

From inside my closed windowless tent I heard and watched Thangboché come alive in the morning. Before light, along with the low hum of monks chanting their morning prayers came the sound of horns and cymbals. Then, with the light came the clanging of yak bells as the animals assembled for their daily loads. A beam of sunlight hit low against my tent and I followed a parade of yaks in silhouette marching across the tent wall on their way further up the mountain.

We'd be following soon, but first we had an important privilege and responsibility to tend to. The Rimpoché, head lama of the monastery and of the entire Khumbu region, had granted us an audience to give his blessing for a safe expedition. We were led into a courtyard off the main temple where we took off our shoes before entering a small square stone room with benches all around and a stove in the middle. It was dimly lit by a window covered with a dark red curtain. After a few minutes of complete silence, the Rimpoché entered the room wearing a red robe with a bright orange shawl. He sat cross-legged in the corner on an orange cushion and said a prayer as he picked up small lengths of red string, wrapping each one around his finger three times and then making a knot. One by one we went before him and offered the prayer shawls which the monastery had given us. He blessed them and put them back over our shoulders. He handed each of us one of the knotted strings that we were to tie around our necks and leave in place for the entire expedition. Though Buddhism was not my religion, in this room, among these mountains, the ceremony seemed exactly right, and I welcomed the lama's prayers. He clapped his hands and the austere ceremony was over, except for giving out a prayer page that he ripped off a pad and handed to us one by one as we left.

The Rimpoché had welcomed us, the invaders, but two years earlier invasions had taken their toll. In the name of progress the monastery had been wired for electricity, and the next day the five-hundred-year-old structure, since rebuilt, burned to the ground. There are two explanations: Circuit overload is the quick answer that doesn't make anyone uneasy. But if you look at the big picture, the Tibetan answer becomes the obvious one: The gods didn't want it.

Frank was actually polishing his shoes when I came into the teahouse for lunch at Deboché. The backside of the Thangboché plateau gets no drying sunshine, and the wide dirt trail has become a steep mudslide oozing all the way down to Deboché. Many desperate grabs at tree roots and branches saved me from the challenge that was now facing several of my companions: removing large quantities of mud from skin and clothes with only small quantities of water.

Deboché has a Shangri-La quality to it—a sheltered garden of trees, flowers, and birds surrounded by tall mountains. We had slid down six hundred feet to get here and now would climb two thousand feet to our next destination, Pheriché, at an altitude of fourteen thousand feet. That's a threshold elevation for the start of serious altitude problems and, after a net gain of fourteen hundred feet today, we'd need a rest day there.

My steps were more deliberate now as I ascended into the thinner air of the high Himalayas. Narrow rocky trails twisted around precipitous ledges with shear drops to thin ribbons of turbulent water far below. The slopes were brown, covered with moss and low bushes. And yet, as I approached the next village, I could see that people have carved out a place to live here. The lower slopes are terraced, albeit narrow and steep, and there are rows of small stone huts, neatly arranged. I passed under a farmer who was working his crop suspended from a rope.

The "mayor" of Pangboché served me tea. I was looking for his brother, Nima Tashi, and he was doing all he could to find him for me. Nima Tashi was a locally renowned climber who had appeared in *National Geographic* magazine after summiting Everest twice. About a year ago he took a bad fall. A friend of mine who had climbed with Nima Tashi, got a message from him and asked me to see if I could help. The message had been "I walk no good because I have broken both wrists of my legs."

It turned out Nima Tashi was "out of town" at the moment, planting potatoes in a village where he rented a piece of flat land.

"We send someone, he come to you," the mayor reassured me.

It was an overnight trip. The mayor and I were getting along great, but I wouldn't be able to make conversation that long. Nima Tashi would have to find me. I took my leave and continued on to Pheriché.

"So, Doc, are you ready to buy time-shares here?" John asked me as we sat in front of our tent on the riverbank, looking out over a wide floodplain and the shallow river meandering through it.

"Yeah, what sold me on this place is that dead cow lying in the water and the guy standing next to it washing himself."

"What I really like is the wind," John replied as he zipped his parka all the way up and tied the hood.

Periché is a bleak, windswept collection of six or eight huts, the highest settlement that's inhabited year round, though none of us could figure out why. We were sharing our waterfront property with a herd of yaks who were wandering around and poking their heads into any tent whose owner was careless enough to leave the flap open. The town is also home to an outpost of the Himalayan Rescue Association (HRA), an organization that provides English-speaking doctors during the trekking season to treat altitude-sick hikers as well as local villagers. Since I was a doctor, it seemed like a place I should visit, at least to warm up. My timing was perfect. As I walked in, a wood fire was going and dinner was just being served. The two American doctors, Bill Binder and Matt Reis, were very friendly. I had chicken and fried potatoes and we discussed mountain medicine into the evening around the pot-bellied stove.

There was only moonlight to illuminate cold stone huts and pairs of yak eyes as I worked my way back to the tent I was sharing with John. I told him about my dinner.

He said, "Yeah, that's one of the perks of being the doctor. But my dinner at the teahouse was even better. A Sherpani girl with a runny nose was able to carry five cups of tea to the table at the same time by placing one finger in each one."

Some combination of the altitude, the cold, the desolation of Periché, and the inactivity of a rest day was causing people to come to me with minor complaints magnified by anxiety. Everyone had developed a cough from deep breathing the cold dry air, and there were headaches, upset stomachs, and diarrhea. One of the two climbers who had hiked to the monastery above Namché told me he'd had diarrhea every day since then. He thought the monk put a curse on him. I laughed but saw he was only half-joking. I was suprised at how much reassurance he needed.

Facades of confidence were beginning to crack. I couldn't be sure all the illnesses were minor and, not being immune to the effects of Pheriché myself, I also could have used some reassurance. But I was the doctor, and part of my responsibility was to project an air of confidence that the others could lean on.

The impromptu clinic outside my tent was winding down. I had seen most of my climbing mates as well as several Sherpas. By now I was feeling lethargic and beginning to believe I was sicker than any of the people I had treated. I looked up and saw another Sherpa limping up the trail toward me and thought, Oh, no, not another one.

He tilted to the left as he walked, taking short steps on his left leg and leaning heavily on two ski poles. Nevertheless he made surprisingly rapid progress, and as he reached me he said, "Dr. Ken-Sab?"

Not until then did I realize this was Nima Tashi. He told me his story, half in English and half with Ong-Chu translating. Porters bringing kerosene had tried to cross the Amphu Lapke Pass but thought the descent was too icy. They left their load at the top and turned back. Nima Tashi's village needed the fuel and he volunteered to bring it down. With two forty-five-pound jugs of kerosene strapped to his back he started his descent, but the cans were only half-filled and as he leaned, the liquid sloshed back, throwing him off the mountain. He slid three hundred feet, ricocheting off ice and rocks, and broke both his ankles. He crawled for fourteen hours until he reached a trail where some trekkers found him. He was eventually taken to Kathmandu, where he had two unsuccessful operations on his left ankle. What hurt him the most was not his ankle or his loss of glory but his inability to provide for his wife and three children. He couldn't herd yaks and was barely able to plant potatoes. All he could do was put the sprouts in the ground after his wife dug the holes. He was in great pain just standing.

He was in even greater pain when I tried to work off his left shoe. The chronic swelling of his ankle had stretched the shoe around his foot. Judging by the tightness of the fit and the awful smell when it finally did come off, the shoe had been on for quite a long time. He lay on the ground and as I examined the scarred, swollen ankle, painful with every motion, I asked a long-shot question: "x-rays?"

Nima Tashi nodded his head, said "I go get," and started to get up.

"Wait a minute, where are you going?"

"Pangboché."

But Pangboché was four hours away. No one in the little crowd of Sherpas around us seemed to see a problem with this, but I refused to let him go. To humor me, Ong-Chu agreed to send someone else.

It was refreshing for me to concentrate on someone who was really sick, a Sherpa whom I had just met but already admired.

No one was sick the next morning, so it was time to take on some more altitude. Our next stop would be Loboché, two thousand feet higher up—the biggest one-day gain on the entire route. Sherpas were taking down our tents and loading our supplies. The traveling circus was moving on.

Our campground was looking like the yak pen it was before we arrived.

My duffel bag didn't want to close. As I was taking a break, out of breath from the struggle, a hand reached around from behind me, removed a tuft of yak hair stuck in the zipper, and closed it effortlessly. It was Nima Tashi. In his other hand he held an envelope of x-rays that a Sherpa boy had fetched overnight.

As bad as his ankle looked, his x-rays looked worse. The right ankle had a simple fracture which had healed. The left ankle was not only still broken, it was dislocated. There was no contact between the bones of the foot and the leg, so that with every step the leg was coming down behind the foot. An American with this injury would be in a wheelchair pushed by a lawyer suing the mountain, the kerosene distributor, and anyone else he could think of. But this was Nepal, and Nima Tashi was trying to grow potatoes to feed his family in a land where walking over uneven ground was the only transportation.

He would need an ankle fusion to make the bottom of the leg and the top of the foot into one piece. It would leave him with a stiff foot and a limp but would take away his pain and give him a solid platform on which he could bear weight. He would also need a bath; otherwise even with a mask on I would be unable to perform surgery on that foot.

Ong-Chu was hard pressed to translate, but when combined with a series of drawings and demonstration limps, the idea came across. One-year-old dislocated ankles are not something an American surgeon sees very often. My plan was to bring Nima Tashi to New York. I felt certain my hospital would donate the necessary services and that climbing friends of Nima Tashi could come up with the airfare. The surgery would be difficult and the long recovery meant that he would have to stay in the States about six months. I asked him which two seasons would be the best to be away. He said it didn't matter; he wasn't doing anything here anyway.

So maybe progress isn't all bad. I have access to a world of modern technology where Nima Tashi's leg could be fixed. Nuclear isotope studies, computerized axial tomography, and major surgery with bone grafting and joint arthrodesis could turn his life around. I could take Nima Tashi into the future, do the surgery, and bring him back. So maybe the Tibetan gods didn't have it right completely, or maybe it was they who brought me here.

I was now the embodiment of his hope, and he escorted me to the edge of town (a distance of three huts) lifting one ski pole to wave good-bye as I left. The trail wound along the flat and sometimes wet floodplain. I soon caught up to the others just before the start of a long uphill slog.

"Come on, Doc," John said, "I'll race you to Loboché."

"Okay," I replied. "The first one there gets a headache," a humorous but effective reminder to everyone to take it slow.

Personally, I didn't need any reminder since slow was the best I could do anyway, moving up on this boulder-strewn slope against a biting wind. At the top was a collection of austere stone monuments, each with the name of a Sherpa who had died in the mountains. This was the Sherpa Memorial, from which the cold wind seemed to emanate.

Just over the crest, the wind died down and the trail leveled off. This was an obvious spot for weary hikers to rest, but none of us did. The place was too cold or maybe just too depressing, even though none of the names that were there then meant anything to me. That would change in subsequent years. As new monuments with the names of my friends were added, I would feel compelled to stop here and remember.

Four thousand feet ago the river had been tumbling. Two thousand feet ago it was meandering. But now, the cold and altitude had combined, finally, to freeze it to a stop. The trail ended abruptly at the frozen river and we looked in vain for the line of boulders that connected one side to the other. They were submerged. Whenever the wind died, we could hear the gurgling of small rivulets flowing below the surface—a warning that the ice cover was not thick enough to cross over. We detoured higher up the mountain, finding a crossing that was narrower, colder, and safer. Heavy monsoon snows of last season created too much runoff this spring, swelling the river and making the usual crossing impassable. The Sherpas put it more succinctly: "Much snow and sun make big water."

We could smell Loboché before we could see it. Muddy fetid water ran over our boots and on down to the frozen river, leaving a brown stain on the white ice. This stream of mountain runoff was more like an open sewer and as we rounded a final turn, its source came into view: three teahouses and two huts stacked on the slope above us. Loboché must be the Nepali word for cesspool.

Ong-Chu had arrived shortly before me and was already setting up his kitchen. I dropped my pack and went over to investigate. Two cook-boys had just left with large empty water jugs and I followed them. Sure enough, they went down to the stream just below the lowest teahouse to a spot where water pooled and stagnated, and began filling their jugs.

"No, no, no," I interceded, "water no good."

"Yes, is okay," they replied, and by way of reassurance pointed to the sign next to them, clearly written in English, "Drinking Water Here." Directly upstream from the sign, each at the level of the corresponding teahouse, were three outhouses built on stilts and perched over the stream.

Why the doctor couldn't understand a sign written in English was puzzling to the cook-boys, but since I insisted, they walked back with their jugs still empty.

"Ong-Chu, this water is very, very bad."

"I know, Dr. Sab, but there's no other water and I'll boil it a lot."

"Ong-Chu, we can't drink raw sewage no matter how long you boil it. You'll have to collect snow and melt it down."

It's a tedious job that consumes a lot of fuel but he said "yes" right away, immediately redirecting his cook-boys out into the snowfield. They thought it was the funniest thing ever, laughing as they went, falling in the snow, and yelling back jokes for the amusement of the Sherpas watching them.

Snow takes a long time to melt, and at dinner there still wasn't enough to go around. Ong-Chu put out "water for members" (melted snow for expedition members) and "water for Sherpas" (boiled sewage). I would have preferred that nobody drink sewage but Ong-Chu insisted it was all right for his crew, reminding me that they always drank that water when they came to Loboché and they'd go right back to drinking it once I left. Ong-Chu was right. No matter how incomprehensible were the rituals of sanitation that I imposed on him, he was ready and willing to carry them out to protect my fragile flock. I stood ready to help the Sherpas whenever they called on me, but I didn't want to develop a paternalistic attitude. For an interloper like me to try to insulate the Sherpas from their environment would be either naive or arrogant.

Going strictly by schedule, gaining two thousand feet called for a rest day. But Loboché was a seriously dirty place and I was hoping to pull out the next morning if everyone felt okay.

Everyone didn't. In the morning a Sherpa told me Ong-Chu was sick so I paid him a visit.

"Yes, Dr. Sab, but then I threw up and now I feel better."

I told him, "Ong-Chu should stop drinking 'Sherpa water' and start drinking 'member water.'" We both laughed, but I was hoping we weren't bringing any of Loboché's diseases out with us.

To be sure everyone was okay, I wanted our convoy to pull out ahead of me so I dawdled awhile taking in the smells and sights.

I checked my topographic map for the route to our destination, Gorak Shep. Dawa, one of the few Sherpas with us who spoke English, came up from behind. I complained to him how inaccurate our Nepalese maps were.

"You know, Dawa, on these maps, water runs uphill."

"Don't complain, Dr. Ken," he responded. "My country is full of miracles."

Gorak Shep means "Dead Raven"—a name in keeping with the general look of the place, although the only birds we saw were lamergeyers (Himalayan vultures) circling overhead on air currents. They no doubt had their eyes on the tired yaks, or tired climbers, lying below on boulders surrounding the two huts that make up the village. Each settlement along the route had had fewer huts than the one before. The last two weren't even villages. They were shelters, like shepherds' huts, used only in the spring and fall when yaks and trekkers come up to graze and drink tea together.

Gorak Shep is the end of the line—the last outpost of "civilization." The trail stops here because for the Sherpas, there's no reason to go higher. They feel instinctively what Western scientists figure out with measurements—any higher altitude is incompatible with sustained life.

From this point on, the Sherpas are here only because we are here. Some few of them share our spirit of adventure. More of them come with us because it's a good job opportunity. The vast majority aren't here at all, because it makes no sense (why go over the top of a mountain when it's so much easier to go around it?) and because the high peaks are where the gods live.

The name Gorak Shep was branded into my memory at a very early age when I read about the first ascent of Mount Everest. It came to symbolize for me the last place on earth—a jumping-off point into the unknown. What would that little boy think now, seeing himself inside that book and about to jump off into that mysterious realm? Just to put one foot across the threshold would make the trip worth it, for both of us.

CHAPTER

3

The only access to Everest is by walking between the mountains on the frozen river which drains its slopes. When it flowed it was called the Dudh Kosi River but at this altitude, frozen to a thickness of fifteen hundred feet, it's called the Khumbu Glacier. Our team started out together along a ravine for a short distance then one by one, we stepped distinctly off the land—the shoreline—and on to the ice. I was entering the frozen realm of Everest, crossing for real that long-ago frontier of my mind.

The yaks seemed to know where they were going and we followed. They led us through a bizarre landscape of gravel slopes and boulders scoured off the mountain but unable to fall to the bottom as sediment since the river was frozen. Instead the rocks accumulated on top, covering the surface of the glacier like a carpet and piling up in endless mounds that tiny humans must surmount one by one.

The glacier is frozen but it still flows. The enormous pressure of the ice liquifies the lower layers and the whole thing slides slowly downhill. Years from now the sediment that we walked on will empty out from the Ganges River and fall to the bottom of the Indian Ocean.

That will be none too soon for me. It was exhausting walking three steps up and sliding two steps back. Sometimes one step up and three steps back. The yaks were better at this than I was, and soon the constant music of the yak bells faded away ahead of me. By now our group had gotten strung out on one side or another of every mound of rocks and I found myself walking alongside Margo with no one else in sight.

Because the glacier moves constantly, the landscape changes enough from year to year so that the route used last season doesn't exist anymore. The first Sherpas to come through each spring mark a new route by piling stones one on top of the other at high points along the way. This works better in theory than it does in practice and it didn't take long for Margo and me to get lost. We found a line of rocks that seemed flatter than the ones around it and guessed it was due to yak traffic so we followed it. Our deduction was confirmed when we started stepping in yak dung. This must be how the yaks know the route: They follow the smell of yak dung. Left to our own devices, we were beginning to think like yaks, and we moved like contented cows along the trail for a while.

"You know, Ken, this dung isn't fresh."

This was a brilliant observation, but very anxiety provoking. Margo was right. Suddenly it became obvious to us that we were following a section of trail from a previous year, well preserved by the cold.

The huge scree slope that we had been very happy to circumnavigate by the trail now had to be climbed. From our vantage point at the top we spotted a train of yaks, their bells silenced by the distance but their red collars standing out brightly against the gray rocky landscape.

Released from our anxiety, we found renewed energy to slog up and down the rubble slopes. We got back on track and once again were free mentally to observe this strange land. The uniform carpet of gravel was interrupted in many places by icebergs upthrusted from the glacier and surrounded by frozen blue lakes. Above us loomed boulders the size of small houses, perched on long pedestals of ice. The sun had melted the surrounding surface, leaving only the column of ice under the boulder's shadow. The bases of these frozen golf tees get narrower and narrower until they snap off, bringing the boulders crashing down to start the whole process over again. This surreal world of ice pinnacles and stone statuary was no less than I expected in the antechamber to Everest.

As I moved mechanically, my eyes fixed on each successive barren mound until they were jarred by a locus of bright colors—the multicolored tents of base camp, entirely out of place on the gray rubble that surrounded them. Exotic visitors had landed there, bringing their own habitats and life-support systems to colonize this lunar landscape.

This was my first impression of base camp and it recurred each time I returned, but base camp becomes a city unto itself after I move inside. Preoccupation with daily routine makes life within seem safe, almost comfortable, and the image of an artificial environment in hostile surroundings quickly recedes from consciousness.

Ong-Chu handed me a cup of tea as I sat on a boulder in the middle of our camp. Each year, each expedition stakes out its own area on the undulating upward-sloping glacier; advance teams were at work with picks and shovels leveling the ice and rubble wherever possible to create platforms for tents and huts. This year there were twelve expeditions with a total of about two hundred people, all with the goal of getting themselves or their neighbors to the summit of Everest. A one-industry town was being built.

As is true for many other towns, base camp is where it is because it's a transshipment point, just like a port or railroad terminus where one mode of transportation must be switched to another to continue the journey. We'd come along the Khumbu Glacier to its source—the massive base of Everest. Just upstream from here the glacier abruptly becomes an icefall as the snow and ice tumble down Everest's slopes like a slow-motion waterfall spilling into the glacier. Base camp is the last stop for the yaks, which can't go any higher. Equipment and supplies have to be off-loaded here, transferring the cargo from four-legged bearers on hooves to two-legged bearers on crampons.

Thirsty as I was, I needed air more than water and could manage only small sips of hot tea between big deep breaths of thin air. We were at seventeen thousand five hundred feet, the bottom of Everest but already far higher than any point in the contiguous United States. Air pressure is only half what it is at sea level, so lungs have to work twice as hard to pull in the oxygen they need.

While I alternated breathing and drinking, I looked around at lots of smiling Sherpa faces. Some had hiked in with us. Others had been here for weeks preparing the camp. They had done a good job. Our camp was placed high up on the glacier—only the Spanish camp was higher—close to the start of the icefall and above most sources of potential contamination of our water supply. Various ledges had been carved into the slope to allow for small groupings of tents to be placed here and there above the natural basin around which the camp was centered and in which the cook tent, mess tent, and future medical tent were situated. The outhouse was placed on the far side of our slope, over the "continental divide" so that any runoff through the glacier would carry down into uninhabited domain.

With my breathing slowed and my thirst quenched, the last few yards from the boulder up to my tent no longer seemed insurmountable. I hiked up and even had enough energy left to remove the foam mat and sleeping bag from my duffel, laying them inside on the tent floor. That was a maximum effort and I collapsed on my back with my feet out the door, unable to bring them in for the moment, since I needed to rest before I could take off my hiking boots.

It was quiet and I was alone in my room. Each of us had his or her own tent at base camp—a necessary island of privacy on a long expedition like this. When I finished staring at the ceiling and felt like my legs had been out of the tent long enough, I unlaced my boots and brought my feet inside, followed, in stages, by my two duffel bags and my backpack. Little by little I was settling into my new home.

Organization was the key. I put one duffel bag on each side of my sleeping bag and took out for easy access: sacks of snack food, two books (one a philosophical treatise, the other a spy novel—depending on my mood), a short-wave radio, a headlight, and a journal to record my thoughts. Within arm's reach I kept a pee bottle, and as far across the tent as possible I put my plastic bag filled with dirty underwear and socks. In arranging my things, I came across a surprise note from Josiane. It turned out to be the first of many she had hidden in my clothes and gear. I made no methodical search for the others, preferring to come across them at unexpected moments.

A rolled-up pile jacket served as my pillow. Next to it I placed a few family pictures and a set of tiny stuffed dolls that Josiane made for me, each one representing a family member so I'd have everyone with me the whole time I was away. My doll stayed at home with my family—to be reunited when I returned. The tent would be my refuge, not only from the harsh physical world but also from the constant and sometimes overpowering social environment around me.

As much as I tried to ignore it, a rock was intruding on my thoughts and on my back. An air mattress which I had laboriously inflated and placed under my foam mat and sleeping bag to insulate me from the ice was not cushioning me from the rubble. Reluctantly I left the comfort of my sleeping bag to go outside while it was still light to smooth out my platform. The tent was held down with rope stays attached to the frame and anchored to large rocks around which slipknots were tied. By undoing two of the knots I was able to reach under the tent floor and remove the offending stone. I redid the knots and got back in to enjoy my much-improved sleeping accommodations, but before I could catch my breath, I heard a loud repeated clang and a Sherpa calling out, "Soup ready!" Maybe the soup was ready, but I wasn't. I would have preferred to stay in my tent and rest but that would give the impression that I was sick and lead to a lot of well-meaning solicitation which would be more tiresome than getting out of my tent now.

"Soup ready" is the Sherpa equivalent of "Come and get it," and the accompanying *clang* was our dinner bell—the result of a spoon being banged repeatedly against an empty oxygen cylinder suspended from a rope outside the mess tent. We filed in wearing our dinner attire: down parkas, gloves, and boots. The sun had disappeared for the day behind some mountain (dominating though they were, I was, as yet, unable to name any of the majestic peaks that surrounded my new neighborhood) leaving us to the ice-cooled afternoon winds that refrigerate this valley.

Outside your own sleeping bag, the warmest place in camp is the mess tent, provided you get a spot near the single propane heater in the corner. The tent was a large half-cylinder dome high enough to stand up in and supported by semicircular ribs of aluminum tubing. Inside was the triumph of two stonemasons brought up from Pangboché: A large flat dinner table pieced together from cut stones and shaped into a neat sharp-cornered rectangle. Parallel to the table on either side were lower stone rectangles covered with foam mats that served as benches. Like any home, the dining area is the social center as well.

"So where's your tent, Ken?" Mike asked.

"Actually, I've got quite a prestigious location on a cul-de-sac overlooking the ice field. Beautiful mountain view."

"Figures. You're the doctor. My tent's got a view of the outhouse."

Dinner was spaghetti and yak burgers served with carrots and tomatoes. Since our yak train would be leaving tomorrow, Ong-Chu was taking advantage of the situation now to provide us with fresh meat and vegetables. Not that one of our loyal cargo transporters had been butchered on the spot. Buddhist law prohibits any animal sacrifice above the Thangboché Monastery, so the yaks were safe here for the time being. But Thangboché was just a few days away, so the meat and vegetables were still fairly well preserved and edible. "Edible," of course, is a relative term. I noticed I wasn't the only one to bite into a yak burger and then quickly empty the contents of my mouth into a napkin.

Todd had been in camp two weeks already, along with Vern Tejas, another of our climbers and the last one for me to meet. Vern was an Alaskan mountain guide and a violinist—the only violinist I ever met who shaved his head and wore a red beret. He was also the only person ever to have climbed Mount McKinley solo in the winter. This was an accomplishment impossible to verify since no one in his right mind was willing to go along with him, but with one look I could appreciate his strength and his intensity and know for sure that he had really done it.

Vern had been supervising the Sherpas and, along with route finders from other expeditions, probing the icefall looking for the best way through it. Everyone was eager to hear what he and Todd had to say.

"The route's pretty direct this year," Todd said, "but it goes close to the west shoulder so there's lots of movement and avalanches."

"A pair of Indian climbers had to turn back today," Vern added. "An eighty-foot hole opened up where there used to be a crack in the ice you could jump across."

The tent door unzipped and in came a cook-boy with dessert. The meals were prepared in the Sherpa kitchen and then delivered over to us. Ong-Chu had attempted to make a cherry cheesecake from a mix. It sounded a lot better than it tasted. After the cook-boy left, some of us slipped out briefly to feed the yaks.

Todd continued, "There are twenty-five ladder sections, none more than five ladders across, at least not yet. There are three vertical walls—one with a slight overhang."

"That's the 'sporty' part," Vern volunteered, "but don't worry, it may collapse before any of you actually get to climb it."

The icefall is only the first 2,000 feet of the route to the summit. At the top of it is Camp I and the start of the Western Cwm—a more gradual upsloping glacier that runs for another 2,000 feet and ends at Camp II. From there, the route goes 5,000 more feet up the sheer face of Lhotse, the fourth highest mountain in the world. Camp III is placed halfway up. After a sideways traverse, we reach the shoulder between Lhotse and Everest (the South Col) where we'll place Camp IV. The climb finishes with a 3,000 foot ascent of the pyramid that forms the summit of Everest.

The cook-boy came back to clear the dishes. Ong-Chu would be pleased that the dessert plates were wiped clean.

I stumbled back to my tent in the dark, having forgotten to bring my headlight to dinner. The air was still, carrying the sounds of the mess tent so clearly I felt I was still inside. Around me, moon glow backlit the camp forming sharp shadows on the ground and turning the ice slopes into a pale blue frozen sea. The sky was intensely black, filled with more stars than I had ever seen before. If no humans belong here, why is this place so beautiful?

Despite the loud sound of Mike's snoring coming from the tent next to mine, I fell into a deep, restful sleep. At this elevation, it's common to have difficulty sleeping but, at least in my case, my fatigue overwhelmed the altitude. Just before sunrise two Sherpas came to my tent with "bed tea," a very pleasant holdover from the days of British colonial rule. Sitting up in my sleeping bag, I left the door flap open, sipped my tea, and watched the sharp shadow of the mountain behind me slowly recede up the glacier, moving silently toward my tent. Soon I would have my personal sunrise.

Outside in the camp, people were stirring. The noise of pots was coming from Ong-Chu's kitchen. Sherpas were rearranging stones around the tents. Yaks were wandering around, eating corrugated boxes and licking the glue. A young Sherpani girl poked her head out of the Sherpa's tent where she had spent the night. After several furtive glances she slipped out and quickly crossed back to her own tent.

The quiet sounds were interrupted by the snorting of a yak. I was struck by the similarity of that noise to the noise of Mike's snoring. After several more sips of tea, the realization gradually came to me that I had been falsely accusing Mike the whole night. High altitude slows thinking; maybe my head wasn't quite as clear as the air.

The sharp shadow line rippling over the stones had almost reached my tent. I was determined to wait until it passed me so I could get up in the sunlight but it was not to be.

"Dr. Sab, Dr. Sab!" came a voice from just outside my tent. Two Sherpas were kneeling outside my door, one with a bloody finger, the other his interpreter. He had caught his finger between two rocks and crushed the tip. Even from inside the tent I could see the injury wasn't serious. Had he been an American, I would have told him to wash it off and put a band-aid on but that wouldn't translate well between cultures. Being careful to avoid any impression that Sherpas might get lesser treatment than members, I came out of my tent, did a thorough examination, cleaned the finger, and put on the band-aid. My patient, as well as his interpreter, left thankful and satisfied.

Over breakfast we watched the yaks being loaded up for their return journey. The Sherpanis are leaving today also. Dawa remarked, "It's not good to have girls in base camp." I recalled the Sherpani girl I had seen this morning scurrying back to her own tent and understood what Dawa meant.

It started to snow just before the yaks and porters and women left. Not heavily, but enough to make the yak drivers anxious to get going before the snow obscured the glacier trail. We weren't going anywhere today, or for the next few days either. We needed time to organize supplies, check equipment, and above all, acclimatize.

The body responds immediately to thin air by increasing the rate of breathing as well as the volume of air taken in. This is what we call being "out of breath." The body compensates for a low concentration of oxygen by increasing the quantity of air that passes through the lungs. After a while, this becomes a losing proposition. The muscle power needed to breathe rapidly and deeply will use more energy than it creates. The long-term response to thin air is to increase the number of oxygen-carrying red blood cells, the amount of enzymes which transfer the oxygen to the tissues, and the number of mitochondria, microscopic factories where the oxygen is actually burned. These changes, collectively called acclimatization, make the body more efficient but still not efficient enough to prevent slow deterioration at this altitude, which is why nobody lives here.

Going higher now would be fatal. The idea is to use the stimulus of thin air at base camp to bring about maximum acclimatization, then climb and get out before the body deteriorates too far. Changes of acclimatization take days to weeks to be completed, so while our bodies are working desperately to catch up, we are taking rest days, organizing the camp and getting used to our new home and to each other.

Doing all she could to make us feel at home was Liz Green, Pete's wife and an Outward Bound wilderness instructor. She had volunteered to come to base camp to act as our camp manager and, not incidentally, to be with Pete. She was also our social interface with the Sherpas.

"I need a volunteer to take a shower," Liz said as she approached us.

"I'll go with you," John said hopefully.

"No, that's not what I meant. Ong-Chu thinks he's got the thing working but we need someone to test it out."

John went off with Liz anyway. I went off to the three-meter dome tent that I would have to turn into a medical facility. The floor was covered with my four yak-loads of medical supplies, most of them in plastic bags and everything neatly labeled. There were also two stacks of oxygen cylinders in wooden crates and between them, on the floor, a Sherpa was sleeping. The supplies would all have to be inventoried, checked for damage, and then arranged.

I was especially anxious to uncrate the oxygen tanks. Oxygen is a precious, and very expensive, commodity on the mountain. Our tanks were made of a thin layer of titanium and prone to leaks or explosions but we were using them because they were lightweight, only seven pounds each. Because of their fragility, it was illegal to have them in the United States. They had to be shipped directly here from a factory in Russia.

The empty crates would be useful for organizing my supplies. I was less sure what to do with the sleeping Sherpa, so I went to find Pete, our diplomat. He had just caught up with us and with his wife. All our equipment had gotten through customs and the interior minister was still alive. If Pete could pull that off, he should have no trouble handling a sleeping Sherpa.

Meanwhile the snowfall got heavier. The test shower was cancelled. The yak drivers quickly finished loading and started off. I ducked into the mess tent. Todd and Vern were in the back surrounded by piles of climbing gear and food. They were weighing out Sherpa loads: each one should be twenty kilos—the standard load for a Sherpa going through the icefall.

"This one's only seventeen kilos," Todd said as he hung it on a fish scale suspended from the tent frame. "What is this, your pack, Vern?"

"Listen, Todd, you'll have to empty it out to make it equal to one of yours."

With a practiced hand, Vern felt the weight of two sacks of rice and gave one to Todd, who added it into the backpack. Twenty kilos exactly.

"Let's see now," Todd said as he took a marker and started making calculations on a paper bag. "We've got fourteen

Sherpas carrying loads. At twenty kilos each, that's two hundred eighty kilos a run. With every third day a rest day, in five days we can have one thousand kilos through the icefall."

Though Todd had once been a high school physics teacher, even he couldn't factor in the effects of bad weather, injuries, and crevasses. The icefall wouldn't be as predictable as Todd's arithmetic, but the plan looked good, at least when written on a paper bag. Our Sherpas would be moving through the icefall tomorrow. My responsibility would be to have the medical tent ready to function by then if necessary.

"Todd, I'm going to need more oxygen crates to get fully organized. Where are they?"

"They seem to disappear as soon as we open them. Everyone's got a use for them. I think Ong-Chu has a few in the kitchen. Gopal [one of our strongest climbing Sherpas] took one for a card table."

John and Mike were sitting with me in the mess tent. Ong-Chu always kept a jug of hot tea available and it was a good place, the only place, to hang out.

"We'll help you round them up."

"Okay, great. We'll declare a general amnesty and see how many we can get back."

All day wasn't enough time to get the medical tent in shape. I used the six crates I had, plus two more that John and Mike had talked the Sherpas out of, but a few more would have been better. I could have pulled rank on Ong-Chu but he was using his crates as tables for the kitchen burners and he needed them as much as I did.

I learned my lesson that first year. In later years I brought along collapsible vinyl shoe racks that opened up into cubby holes. They were fastened onto poles jammed down into the ice under the tent floor. That way the Sherpas could keep their crates.

My crates were laid sideways and stacked around the periphery of the tent to act as shelves, each stack held together with duct tape. Supplies were arranged on the shelves according to function.

I had eight different kinds of antibiotics. Since I would be unable to take any cultures, the cause of any infection would always be uncertain and if my best guess didn't work I'd have to be able to fall back on another. Plus, who knows who's going to be allergic to what.

There was a whole spectrum of painkillers. Everything from IV morphine and Demerol to analgesic hemorrhoid pads. For any digestive problem—upset stomach, nausea, vomiting, constipation, diarrhea—I had the pills. I had treatments for chronic cough and for asthma, for all eye, ear, nose, and throat problems. I had medications for skin conditions, from a fungus infection to a third-degree burn.

I had to treat every climber from head to toe, from a fractured skull to athlete's foot. In planning what to bring, I had compiled a list of every possible injury or disease I might encounter and, for each one, made a separate list of every item needed to treat it step by step. If I didn't bring it, I wouldn't have it and would have no chance of getting it. But I couldn't bring everything. Weight, volume, and "usability" on the mountain all have to be considered. Pills, yes; but what about liquids? They're heavy and bulky and they would all freeze; could they be defrosted? If they were, how would they work? Simple surgical instruments, yes; but what about a cardiac defibrillator? If a climber needed that, he was probably going to die anyway, so it wasn't worth all the extra pounds.

Perhaps even harder were the decisions about the quantities to bring. IV fluids, for example, are very heavy. Should I bring enough to treat one person for shock for one day or enough to treat my entire team for one week? What about the other teams on the mountain? Many of them didn't have doctors. I wouldn't turn away a sick or injured climber no matter where he's from, nor would I withhold my limited supplies from anyone who needed them. But how do I balance that against my responsibility to provide for my own teammates?

I'd have to make practical decisions all along the way, consider the odds, and resign myself to the idea that disasters might occur that I would not be equipped to handle, either because I didn't have the equipment, or, far harder to accept, because I didn't have the skills.

People die easily here. I wasn't sure of my ability to treat life-threatening conditions caused by high altitude, and my uncertainty weighed heavily on my mind. Though I'd climbed as high as twenty thousand feet and taken care of many mountain emergencies, Everest is a special case. Conditions are extremely harsh and it was likely that some of the most serious illnesses I'd confront would be ones I've never seen before. Everyone presumed that I'd be able to handle any emergency and I encouraged that belief by projecting an air of confidence, but the specter of a climber dying because I didn't know how to save him gave me an extra reason to be uncomfortable here.

It got dark in the tent and without my asking, a Sherpa came in to hang a lantern. I continued a while longer but I was tired and short of crates. I left the tent with piles of supplies still scattered on the floor, but at least the itinerant Sherpa from this morning had been assigned another place to sleep.

I was awakened by a metallic clang and was glad it wasn't for me. The Sherpas were getting up to go through the icefall but, at least this time, I could stay in my sleeping bag, warm and tired. A light suddenly went on outside—someone had lit a fire in the *lhapso* altar and soon juniper smoke was wafting into my tent. No one enters the icefall without first being blessed by the sacred smoke. The rumbling noise of boots on gravel told me the Sherpas were leaving, and then all was quiet again. The fire in the lhapso burned down but the light didn't go out. As long as our climbers were on the mountain the fire would be tended—the candle in the window would burn.

A few hours later I was out of my tent in the pre-dawn light admiring the scene. I was beginning to know the neighborhood: Snow glistened on the west shoulder of Everest as it sloped downward to the Lo Lha Pass, behind which I could see the mountains of Tibet. Surrounding me on three sides were well-constructed stone walls, and below, each of my feet rested on a solid slab of rock. Between them was a deep blue hole chopped out of the glacier. No outhouse in the world had a better view, but it was cold and I didn't want to hang around too long. I wedged the roll of toilet paper back between the stones and returned over the ravine.

Three climbers were waiting for me outside my tent. Two weren't even from my camp. It was morning sick call. The first was a German guy with hemorrhoids. His expedition had no medical help but he had heard there was a doctor with the Americans. He came with a translator who took advantage of the situation to ask me about his own diarrhea. The third was Pinzo, one of our Sherpas. I recognized him by the red baseball cap he always wore.

"Dr. Sab, I have pain here and here," he said, pointing to his back and neck.

"How long?"

"Six years."

There was no way I was going to diagnose and treat somebody with six years of back pain this morning here on the Khumbu Glacier, but he didn't know that, and telling him would be the same as saying, "Get lost." So I took out my medical kit and went through a full examination, doing a lot of irrelevant tests, not even knowing what I was looking for. When I felt that he felt it had gone on long enough, I nodded my head knowingly, put away my instruments, and gave him a little packet of anti-inflammatory pills. I figured it couldn't hurt, and if he had chronic muscle strain it might even help.

Ong-Chu spotted me coming down the slope to the mess tent. He knew why I was late for breakfast and was only too eager to make me a special order of cheese omelette and fried potato. There was a jug of hot water, a bar of soap, and a towel set up on a rock outside the mess tent now and I washed up while I waited. Although everyone had finished eating, they were hanging around to enjoy the morning sun.

There was a rumor that the shower was working.

"Listen everybody," Liz said, "there should be enough time for three people to shower this morning."

"Okay," said Mike, trying to get things organized quickly. "I'll go with Liz and Margo."

"Sorry, Mike, the showers will be consecutive not concurrent. The problem is deciding who the three dirtiest people are."

I guess I was one of them. I got the third tee-off time, ten-thirty. Climbing Everest is one thing, but taking a shower late in the morning is really living dangerously. At this time of year clouds move upvalley early, and by afternoon the entire sky is overcast. The only (more or less) reliable sunshine comes the first few hours after sunrise. Taking a chance on drying in the sun after that gets risky.

The shower was another three-walled stone structure with a blue tarp over the top and down the front. On a pole in the center was a ten-gallon jug with a spigot and a rubber tube. A cook-boy stood ready, and when you yelled, "Yes, water," he brought a bucket of hot water from the kitchen, climbed a ladder and poured the water into the jug. It actually worked pretty well. Even though the shelter was drafty, the trickle of water kept me warm if I turned continuously. I soaped up and rinsed off and then tried to wash my hair a second time since it still didn't feel clean. That was a mistake. The water ran out and I stood wet in the cold air with a head full of soap, yelling, "Yes, water! Yes, water!" By the time the cook-boy responded with another bucket of water, contact with the rocks had turned my feet blue.

The shower was a success. For a few minutes I was able to shed my multiple layers of clothes from top to bottom and let my skin breathe. I felt clean and mentally refreshed. As I came out from under the tarp I noted with relief that the clouds were still far downvalley.

With twelve expeditions on the mountain and nearly every one speaking a different language, going from camp to camp was like touring an Olympic village. There was generally a lot of camaraderie between the groups, but with so many nationalities intensely focused on the same goal, conflicts were bound to occur. After lunch Todd was heading for a meeting of group leaders at the British camp and he asked me to come along. I had planned to finish organizing the medical tent but I still didn't have any more crates to work with, and anyway I had spent the whole day there yesterday and could use a change of scene.

"The Spanish are shitting in our water!" was the first thing I heard as we entered the tent. Rob Hall, the New Zealand team leader, was complaining. "That's why we're getting so many cases of dysentery."

I recognized Rob right away. We had met in Antarctica six years ago during a whiteout—a weather condition in which stirred-up surface snow and fog combine to eliminate visibility. I was treating a member of my team for severe frostbite. I could hardly see my hand in front of my face but Rob, on a different team, was able to make his way over to our camp and lead the injured climber out. Seeing him for the first time since then, it was as if he had suddenly emerged from that fog into which he had last disappeared. After a big hello and a warm hug, I took a seat on a supply box.

Representatives from almost all the expeditions were sitting around a long folding table, sipping tea. Only the Russians were missing. It looked like a meeting of the U.N., with English as the official language.

"Perhaps you could move your latrine," suggested the British group leader, who was trying to moderate the discussion. Because the Spanish were the highest up on the glacier, their water ran down through everyone else's camp. We were the next ones down but it wasn't a problem for us since we drew our water from a long hose that collected runoff well above all the camps.

"What are we going to do about the Russians climbing the wrong route? Their permit is for the South Pillar but they're doing the South Col."

To prevent overcrowding, the Nepalese limit the number of permits issued for any one route. The South Pillar is much tougher than the South Col, so it's tempting for an expedition to veer onto the easier climb.

"It's not just the Russians. Everyone's taking the South Col route." And with that, a lot of dirty looks passed around the table.

Todd leaned over to me: "This could work to our advantage. The Russians are a strong team. If they put in fixed lines on the Lhotse Face, it will save us a lot of work."

"I think we should turn the Russians in," said an angry voice with an Indian accent. "They'd be banned for five years."

"That won't do any good," came the reply. "Russians just change their names and come back with different passports."

The British leader hung up a blackboard. "We've got to work out a maintenance schedule for the icefall."

We had already heard from Todd and Vern that the icefall was especially tumultuous this year. The pressure of the ice opens and closes crevasses, crumpling some ladders and leaving others suspended in space; it causes avalanches which bury fixed ropes (ropes which are anchored to the ice) and sections of trail. All the expeditions would be moving repeatedly through the icefall over the next two months and needed to cross as quickly and safely as possible each time. It made sense to share the continuous burden of maintaining the route. Larger expeditions would be responsible for longer periods but each expedition would have a turn, using its own equipment and personnel. One leader, however, confided in Todd that he didn't think some expeditions were capable of maintaining the icefall.

The schedule, blocked out on the blackboard, was erased and rewritten several times until most of the grumbling subsided. As we left the meeting, Todd was pleased.

"The icefall starts to really break up the first two weeks in May," he told me. "That's when it requires the most maintenance, but it's also the time when most successful summit attempts are made and when it's most important to conserve your resources for higher up. We've got no icefall responsibility those two weeks."

When we got back to camp one of our Sherpas gave me an effusive greeting. "Thank you, Dr. Sab, for all your help. I feel much better now."

"You're welcome," I replied as I shook his hand. "I'm glad I could help you."

As he left, I turned to Todd with a question: "Who is that guy?"

It was Pinzo—the Sherpa with six years of back pain. He didn't have his red baseball cap on. Sherpas don't change clothes very often, and before we get to know them as individuals we tend to identify them by what they're wearing. I didn't recognize him without the cap. The improvement in his condition may have been due to the pills but more likely was just from the relief of having somebody pay attention to his complaint for the first time in six years.

The gourmet cuisine that night was boiled potatoes, Spam, and beans, accompanied by updates on everyone's symptoms. One person started it going and that reminded all the others. Even Koncha, the cook-boy, joined in with a complaint of a headache. I made a sortie to the medical tent to count out pills for my patients. Each allotment was carefully wrapped in toilet paper to maintain "sterility," sealed with tape, and labeled with the climber's name. Back at the mess tent, I distributed the personalized packets of toilet paper including one of aspirin for Koncha, who was delighted I hadn't forgotten him. By then dinner was over. Not only had the food been lousy but I hadn't even had a chance to eat it. I finished the evening wondering if that last thought made any sense at all.

CHAPTER
4

My tent was being shaken to wake me up. Ong-Chu was outside yelling, "Dr. Sab, Dr. Sab!" This kind of intrusion was pretty daring for a Sherpa, so I knew there must be a big problem.

"Come quick, come quick. Kitchen-boy very sick."

I dressed quickly—I was sleeping with two-thirds of my clothes on anyway—and got out of the tent. The predawn air was still and cold. Ong-Chu was in front of me, backlit by the dim light that reflected off the towering ice walls surrounding the camp. His eyes were intensely focused on me, but I had to pee before I could do anything else. Ong-Chu watched and waited while I did, impatiently shifting his weight from one foot to the other, then hurried me over the snow to the cook tent.

In the yellow glare from the propane heater, I saw the kitchen boy lying on a mat on the floor. It was his usual sleeping spot, but this morning Ong-Chu had been unable to awaken him. With a sinking feeling I realized this was Koncha—the one who had complained to me last night about a headache, and whom, in the midst of everyone else's complaints, I had simply treated by giving aspirin.

He was unconscious, with his eyes closed, writhing around on the floor and moaning. From across the tent I could hear rales—bubbling sounds coming from his lungs. He didn't respond to his name or anything else except painful stimulation. When I pushed my knuckles hard into his sternum, it caused him to change the pitch of his moans and make a vague arm gesture to push me away. His pulse and respirations were rapid and shallow. His skin was clammy and pale.

Our entire Sherpa crew had gathered in the tent, silently watching the examination. Now that I had finished, they all looked toward me, waiting to be told what to do. I recognized the signs. This was end-stage high altitude pulmonary edema, which had progressed to include cerebral edema. I was the base camp doctor—the expert—and this was the first case I had ever seen.

Pulmonary edema is a poorly understood condition which strikes climbers suddenly and unpredictably at high altitude. Lungs must remain inflated to function. They're composed of millions of tiny air sacs that stay open as long as the air pressure inside them is high enough to resist the pressure of the blood on the other side of their delicate membranes. Although the exact mechanism is very complex, it's as if the low air pressure at high altitude is no longer adequate to hold back the fluid portion of the blood, which suddenly pours across the membrane like water through a break in a dike. The air sacs fill with fluid and lungs become sponges. Koncha was drowning.

I told Ong-Chu we would have to move him to the medical tent right away. I was annoyed now that I didn't have the tent arranged yet. There were still piles of supplies all over the floor. Just then Pete appeared in the cook tent, grasping the situation right away. I left him to work out the logistics of carrying Koncha over while I went ahead to pick out what I needed from the shelves and off the floor.

Quickly I found the bags of IV fluid, but they were frozen. I took out syringes, needles, catheters, and tape; lined up vials of medications; and then forced myself to stop for a few seconds and picture each scenario that could develop from this starting point and review the steps I would take at each turn. Knowing how to handle each contingency would allow me to work smoothly no matter what happened, and seeing me calm would keep everyone else calm.

Pete came in with Koncha followed by the Sherpas, who cleared a space on the floor, laid Koncha down on two foam mats, propped up his chest, and covered him with a sleeping bag. Someone brought the propane heater from the mess tent. Our *sirdar*, or head climbing Sherpa, Lakpa-Rita, came in with a powerful flashlight, beaming it wherever he thought I was looking. Although it was light outside, the sun wasn't up yet and it was still dark inside the tent.

I listened to Koncha's lungs again, this time with a stethoscope though I hardly needed one. The rales were everywhere. His pulse was 112, nearly twice normal; blood pressure was 90/60, on the low side, but okay; respiration was forty-eight, more than three times normal—he was gasping for air. Oxygen saturation (the percent of oxygen in the blood compared to full capacity) was twenty-six. That was the lowest I'd ever seen. Normal for a Sherpa at this altitude would be in the seventies. In the States, anesthesiologists panic if a patient's rate drops below ninety.

Koncha was still unconscious. Fluid had also leaked into his brain, causing cerebral edema. Similar to what was happening in the lungs, fluid was accumulating within the brain cells, causing them to swell and disturbing the normal electrical pattern which maintained coordination and consciousness.

I started with a dose of dexamethasone, a steroid that draws fluid out of the brain. I had to give it by injection into the muscles, rather than intravenously, since it would take at least fifteen minutes to defrost the IV bag, which had been sent out to the kitchen to be warmed. Putting cold fluid in his veins would only throw him into hypothermia. Pete hooked up an oxygen tank and strapped the mask over Koncha's face. His saturation went up to sixty but then Koncha pulled the mask off. I was glad to see that. His movements were becoming a little more purposeful and coordinated.

Pete replaced the oxygen mask and made sure it stayed there. Sherpas brought the IV bag back from the kitchen. I held it against my face and it seemed warm enough. It was Ringers Lactate, a solution used to treat shock by increasing blood volume. My patient already had too much fluid in him so I would have preferred using a different solution like D5W but I couldn't find any. The bags were still lost on the tent floor somewhere.

Three Sherpas held Koncha down while two more steadied his arm so I could look for a vein to start the IV. I went for the easiest spot, the inside of the elbow, and scored a direct hit with the catheter needle. Koncha squirmed and the blood stopped flowing. I jiggled the needle a bit, got it going again, and taped it in place. Pete made it permanent by tying the whole arm to a polystyrene oxygen cylinder cover.

With two more doses of dexamethasone, as well as several doses of other medications, and continuous 100 percent oxygen, Koncha became alert and fully responsive. His rales quieted down to where I needed a stethoscope to hear them. He was able to take a pill so I gave him two doses of nifedipine—a drug which moves fluid out from the center of the body into the extremities, but can cause a sudden drop in blood pressure. I wasn't worried about that now. His blood pressure had been holding steady and the IV was working well in case I had to get more fluids into him in a hurry. On oxygen, his saturation was in the seventies. Off it, it was in the sixties. He was even holding his own oxygen mask now.

Koncha was dramatically better. He was stable, although pumped up with medication and on high maintenance. I was surprised at how aggressively I had treated him and was really pleased with the rapid response. Still, he would have to be evacuated to a lower altitude. That would be the definitive treatment.

Helicopter rescue is possible at this altitude but the weather has to be perfect. Today there were gusty winds with an overcast sky. He would have to be carried down to the HRA station at Pheriché. That journey would drop him 3,500 feet and his condition should improve considerably once he got there. But Pheriché was at least eight hours away and for the first five there would be hardly any altitude loss. His condition could easily deteriorate en route and I wouldn't be going along. The Sherpas carrying Koncha had to move quickly despite their load and I would only slow them down.

A ladder was rigged up to serve as a stretcher and we placed Koncha sitting semiupright so that the fluids in his lungs would collect at the bottom, leaving breathing passages near the top dry enough for air to flow through. I wrote a long note for the HRA doctors and prepared two syringes of dexamethasone, one for the road and one to be given three hours en route—a point at which I guessed there would not yet be any significant descent and where Koncha might need a little boost.

I watched them go off down the glacier: four Sherpas holding the ladder with Koncha sitting up, his oxygen mask connected by a tube to a tank in the backpack of a Sherpa trailing behind. Other Sherpas followed, carrying additional oxygen. As detail was lost in the middle distance, the cortege began to resemble a pasha touring his kingdom while inhaling from a hookah.

The sky in the background was gray. It occurred to me that Koncha's illness had come on with overcast weather and a falling barometer. His body reacted to the lower air pressure like it had suddenly gained altitude.

A small cheer went up as I entered the mess tent. It was past lunchtime but everyone was still hanging around. Climbers were checking their gear: adjusting harnesses, sealing boot cracks, sharpening crampons. There was talk of doing exercise this afternoon. Acclimatization was catching up to them and they were starting to gain some energy.

"We should go for a hike today," Hugh said to no one in particular.

"Yeah, we should," Mike replied, but he was staring at the tent wall as he spoke.

I didn't want to hear about it. I hadn't thought about climbing all day, hadn't checked my gear, and I was tired. I consoled myself with the idea that neither Hugh nor Mike sounded like they meant it.

I couldn't have gone for a hike even if I wanted to. I had to stay in contact in case the Sherpas needed advice. Once an hour, someone would climb a boulder next to the mess tent and hold an antenna in the air as I angled the receiver back and forth trying for the clearest signal. All afternoon climbers came and went from the bottom part of the icefall while I sat on a rock in base camp. They were exercising, testing their equipment, and practicing ladder crossing— something many experienced climbers, including myself, have never done. Impatiently, I listened to radio reports that progress was slow. Koncha was doing okay, but not great.

The last radio call we were able to receive was from just outside Pheriché where the trail wound around a mountain. The HRA doctors would soon be taking care of Koncha (but it would be several weeks before I found out he made a full recovery). I expressed frustration that we were out of contact but what I really felt was relief. I was secretly glad to lose the signal since it meant I could rejoin my expedition.

In the morning, as I approached the outhouse, I was pleased to see that it had been upgraded. A blue tarp covered what had been the open air entrance. Inside was a bigger surprise. An upside-down oxygen crate with a circle cut out rested over the hole in the ice. It really ticked me off. I'd been looking for the missing crates to arrange the med tent and some jerk had taken one to use for a toilet seat. To add insult to injury, the circle wasn't even cut in the right spot.

The team came to breakfast full of enthusiasm from yesterday's icefall practice. The air was filled with questions about our climbing schedule from here on.

"Who put the oxygen crate in the outhouse?" I asked as I entered the tent.

Either no one knew or no one was admitting it.

"I don't know," John said, "but now at least I can read a magazine in there."

Todd ignored my interruption and began to systematically lay out our climbing plan.

"So far, we've got twenty-eight Sherpa-loads at Camp One. Tomorrow, Pete, Vern, and two Sherpas, Lakpa-Rita and Gopal, will start up to Camp Two. Once we've got our spot there, we'll start moving our loads from One to Two. In three or four days the rest of us should be able to move up to One, take a rest day, move on to Two, sleep over, and then come back down. After a rest we go up again, working our way up to Three this time, then backing off again. Another good rest at base and then we go for the Camp IV summit."

It sounded like a good climbing plan but it was also good medicine. We would be gradually exposing ourselves to higher altitudes for short periods. After each exposure, we'd be moving lower to give our bodies a chance to catch up. As much as possible we'd follow the rule of "climb high, sleep low," but Everest is such a huge mountain, sometimes we'd be forced to climb high and sleep high.

Todd concluded, "It's a good plan but on Everest the only thing that's sure is that things won't go according to plan."

Sitting outside my tent I was enjoying the morning sun and sorting methodically through my gear. I hadn't checked my technical climbing equipment since leaving New York and, with all the distractions here, it felt unfamiliar. I had been looking forward to this time but instead of feeling excited I felt nervous.

Deep in thought, I didn't hear Chuldum approach. "Good morning, Dr. Sab."

Nice of him to come say hello, I thought for a second. But only for a second, realizing right away something else must have brought him here.

"Kima is sick, please. He come back because of bad stomach."

It sounded serious but on further questioning it seemed that Kima had had more than his share to drink yesterday. This was just a chang overdose. I brought him a bottle of Mylanta and told him to drink the whole thing.

As I came out of Kima's tent, a Sherpa from Rob Hall's New Zealand team was waiting for me. He said, "Sherpa sick."

"I know." I pointed to Kima's tent.

"No. Sherpa fell in icefall."

"Bleeding?"

"Yes."

"Where?"

"Yes."

"No, where is he bleeding?"

"In the icefall."

Clearly, I could use more information so I went off to find Rob.

The story was that a Sherpa with the New Zealand team had fallen while descending the lower, "easy" part of the icefall. He was coming down fast, didn't bother to rope up, and tripped over his crampons, falling eighty feet into a crevasse and landing on his head. Though we always try to slow the Sherpas down, they rarely take the time to tie themselves into safety lines since, amongst themselves, the speed at which they can travel through the mountains is a great source of status. Peer pressure prevents them from being safe.

The New Zealand team was sending some climbers up to meet the injured Sherpa, who had already been pulled from the crevasse, and help escort him down. The team had a doctor but she hadn't yet arrived in base camp, so they were looking for medical help.

I could see four dots moving slowly down the icefall and three dots moving rapidly up to meet them. When the dots converged, we got a radio call:

"He's conscious and able to walk but there is a big cut on his head and he's bleeding from his nose. Should we let him continue down under his own power?"

"Yes," I reasoned, "as long as he can walk, it will be quicker and safer."

A few minutes later we got another call:

"We're having trouble. He's bleeding a lot more now and not walking so well."

"Lay him down on a stretcher, compress his nose with something, and make sure he can breathe."

"We're already doing that."

The dots stopped moving for a while and then started down again. They were at least two hours away. I went to the med tent I managed to clean up yesterday and prepared to mess it up again. This wasn't just a nosebleed—I set up for a major emergency. For this one I was more comfortable. There was time to get ready, I was more experienced (two days' worth), my tent was better organized and, being a surgeon, I was more at ease handling trauma.

It sounded like the Sherpa might have an epidural hematoma—a collection of blood under the skull. A severe head injury can cause a blood vessel in the brain to break. At first the victim has a lucid interval—a short time when he feels relatively okay—but as bleeding continues, pressure inside the rigid skull builds up and soon causes compression of the softer brain tissue.

When the rescue team reached the bottom of the icefall we got a call saying that the Sherpa was still bleeding, could no longer talk, and was losing consciousness. We could see them moving rapidly over the moraine just above the Spanish camp, then lost sight of them as they crossed through the camp. We waited. They didn't come out the other side. We waited. They weren't coming out. Skip went up to see what happened. A few minutes later I went up too.

The Spanish team saw the rescuers coming toward their camp. They had no idea what was going on since all the radio contact had been with us, but they had a doctor who waved them in. In the confusion, the rescuers just followed the gesticulating Spaniards and didn't realize they weren't the ones they had been talking to on the radio. Their doctor had stolen my patient.

Taken by surprise, they weren't at all prepared and were now scrambling around looking for IVs and medicines. There were at least ten of them in a tiny tent yelling at each other. The Sherpa was still tied to the transport stretcher, which rested on two crates and took up all of one side of the tent. He looked pretty bad. His face and forehead were edematous and covered with blood, but there was no active bleeding from his nose. His eyes were swollen shut. Three "assistants" were crowding the patient on the only side with access, effectively blocking out the doctor who was still trying to start an IV. On top of that, someone with a big video camera was jockeying for position trying to get close-up shots.

The IV was in but it wasn't working. When the doctor backed up to wait for a fresh needle, I took the chance to talk to him. His name was Ricardo Arreghi and he spoke a little English. I told him we were all set up downstairs and ready to take the patient. The Sherpa had survived a two-hour descent through the icefall; I was sure he could make it another three minutes to our camp. Ricardo wouldn't hear about moving him even though he hadn't been unpacked yet. I really felt the patient would be better off with us rather than in the middle of a Chinese fire drill, but there didn't seem to be any point in starting an ego fight. Ricardo got the IV going, showed me he had a lot of supplies (though they were all still in barrels) and seemed to know what he was doing—though with his limited English it was hard to know for sure. Skip and I felt superfluous and we left. No one noticed.

Putting away supplies and rearranging the medical tent was depressing. I had given a party and no one came. I felt at fault. I had deferred to another doctor despite my better judgment because he had been more forceful.

I reasoned it would be more productive now for me to exercise than to sit stewing about the patient. I said to Skip, "I heard there's a mountain around here," and he said he'd show me where.

It was a short walk from our camp to the start of the icefall but an even shorter walk would have been okay with me. I was out of breath right from the start and stumbled along all the way up to the crampon point—the abrupt line where the spill of the icefall meets the glacial ice and the surface is not yet covered with gray rubble. It's where we have to attach our crampons. Except for just a few notable rock outcroppings, the route from here to the summit is white.

We were not starting for the summit though. I was here with Skip to get a shakedown cruise on the ice. Frank, John, and Mike came along too, not losing a chance to pose as lighthearted experts, having been in the icefall themselves for the first time yesterday.

The initial indication of a climber's skill is how he handles his equipment. Since I was with four people I'd never climbed with before, that thought came immediately to mind as I snapped a crampon onto my boot and caught the tip of my glove in it. As I took my hand out of the glove and then released the crampon to get the glove out, everyone looked on politely.

The sound of crunching snow was reassuring but otherwise I wasn't having much fun. Each step was an effort. I managed to keep up with the group only because they were scampering off from side to side investigating every ice formation like frisky dogs out to play. Meanwhile I was moving as little as possible trying to make every step count.

Luckily for me, this exercise had to end early so I could get back in time for a meeting of doctors the New Zealanders had requested.

"Gee, I'd like for us to stay out longer but I've got to get to that meeting."

Skip said I seemed to get better as I went along but we'd have to leave early when we went through the icefall for real. This was his polite way of telling me I was very slow.

When I arrived at the New Zealand camp, I was surprised to see the injured Sherpa, named Pasang-Nuru, lying in a sleeping bag on a stone table in the middle of the mess tent, connected to an IV suspended from the ceiling. The New Zealand team had brought their Sherpa back and the meeting had been convened to decide what to do next. Besides Ricardo and me, there were three other doctors: a British general practitioner named Peter Davis; an Indian military doctor named Anil Bhagwan; and a Russian anesthesiologist whose name we never got. He was the only one who couldn't speak English.

Despite the obvious difficulties, the group got along well. Each of us did our own examination: Pasang looked worse than before—more swollen, less conscious, his face still covered with dried blood. Ecchymosis (black and blue patches) was developing around his eyes. I forced open the puffy lids to check his retinas with an ophthalmoscope. Swelling of the blood vessels there would indicate a severe pressure buildup in the brain. The vessels were flat. His pupils were equal and reacted to light but the right one reacted slowly, suggesting some increased pressure on the right side.

We sat around the table with the subject of our conversation lying between us. Rob and several Sherpas sat with us, jumping at any chance to be useful. Routinely, they passed around tea and biscuits. Todd came in, took a seat and like the others, waited to help.

There was easy agreement on the treatment plan. We needed to prevent shock by maintaining blood pressure but at the same time had to keep down the brain swelling—and get Pasang evacuated as soon as possible. We considered which supplies we needed and who had what. Each camp contributed equipment and medications. I gave Todd a list and he came back with our propane heater, pulse oxymeter, several IV bags, and a urinary catheter.

Even though Pasang was on full oxygen flow, his oxygen saturation was down around 60 percent. Peter set up an aspirator (a vacuum bottle with a hose and nozzle) that was powered by a foot pump and handed it to the anesthesiologist. He used it to clean out the mouth while a Sherpa pumped the foot pedal. Despite its primitive look, the gadget worked well and oxygen saturation came up into the seventies.

But Pasang was gradually tightening up. His muscles were sporadically becoming rigid and then going into spasm. The Russian made a tight fist and said, "Diazepam." Peter drew up the muscle-relaxing medication but it was a respiratory depressant and I was reluctant to let it be given. To express my concern to our anesthesiologist, I breathed deeply, pointed to the medication and then stopped breathing. He understood but said no, made a fist again, and pointed to the patient. Everyone else was in favor of giving it so I was overruled but I made sure the endotracheal tube and ambu bag were close at hand. The injection relieved the spasms immediately and made no change in the respiratory rhythm. It turned out to be a good move.

From time to time one of us would move around the table to check pupils, pulse, blood pressure, oxygen saturation, urine output, and reaction to stimuli. We adjusted oxygen flow, changed IVs, and emptied the urine drainage bag. It was getting cold even with the dual flames of the propane heater. Sherpas brought in a gas stove, lit both burners, and the tent warmed up some. We now had four open flames in a room where we were pumping oxygen at eight liters per minute, but for some reason the place didn't blow up.

Rob asked the Sherpas to feed everybody. Bowls of noodles and salami were brought in and placed around the periphery of the same table our patient was lying on. Our small talk across the patient on the dinner table was accompanied by a background hum of prayers coming from the Sherpas around us.

Finally radio contact was made with Kathmandu. A helicopter would be coming, but not before morning and then only if the weather was good. We'd have to keep our Sherpa alive through the night but his condition was slowly deteriorating. It was looking more and more like he wouldn't make it. His pulse had sped up to 110, his pressure had dropped to 70/30. Saturation was in the sixties despite full oxygen. Urine output was barely enough to keep his kidneys working. And he had blown a pupil: The pupils were now unequal, with the right one fixed and dilated. He had had a full-blown seizure, losing urine and feces. Pressure was building inside his brain.

His spasms were getting harder and harder to control, even with increasing doses of diazepam, which we were fast running out of. Anil gave an empty cardboard diazepam box to a Sherpa and asked him to go around to all the camps to look for more. He came back a half-hour later with four from the Dutch camp next door. They looked through their medical supplies, matched up the boxes, and gave us all they had.

The next step would be to drill a burr-hole in the skull with a hand tap to relieve the pressure. None of us had ever done it before and we couldn't be sure exactly where to put it. Perhaps sensing our anxiety, Pasang decided to improve. His blood pressure came up to 120/70, his pulse to 100, and saturation to the low eighties. Best of all, his right pupil was again reactive and equal to the left. It now appeared Pasang would live.

The crowd dwindled. Anil and I and two Sherpas agreed to sleep over. Rob wouldn't leave even though there wasn't much he could do. As expedition leader, he felt that his place was here with the sick Sherpa. It was a noble sign of respect for Pasang and loyalty to Sherpas in general—a loyalty that would one day be reciprocated in more dire circumstances far higher on the mountain.

Anil took the first shift. I fell asleep listening to the steady low-pitched drone of prayers coming from the Sherpa tents all around us. The New Zealand camp had a generator to power the lights and Rob left it running all night. He had never done that before and calculated it would probably run out of fuel at about 4:00 A.M. He set his alarm for then and, just a few seconds after it went off, the lights went out. He had calculated too exactly right. While Rob fumbled around in the dark for his headlight, Pasang had another seizure and vomited. It must have been total chaos but Anil handled it so smoothly I slept through the whole thing. At least that's what he told me later. I kidded him that I suspected he had fallen asleep and had a nightmare.

There was no second shift. I was sleeping so soundly Anil decided to continue his watch until morning. At first light I awoke to the same sound to which I had fallen asleep; the Sherpas had been praying continuously. Together we had all brought Pasang through the night.

I went outside to get some air and check the weather. It was calm in the predawn light, perfect for a helicopter landing. I could see some activity in the American camp. Skip and Todd were getting ready to go up the icefall and I walked over to meet them.

"We dodged another bullet," I told Todd.

They were delighted to hear it and relieved for the expedition as well. A death, especially one coming so early on, would rattle the Sherpas, not to mention us, and shake the expedition at its foundation.

The New Zealand tent was filling up again when I got back. In preparation for the helicopter, Peter was tying Pasang to a stretcher and a Sherpa was stuffing all his personal belongings in a knapsack. Pasang was more alert and talking a little bit.

"What's he saying?" I asked one of the Sherpas.

"He's cursing at us for tying him down."

That was a good sign.

The helicopter flew over base camp and the effect was electrifying. All of us stopped what we were doing and turned our heads skyward. People ran toward it as it started to settle down about four hundred yards from the camp in a flat spot which the Sherpas had carved out of the rubble early that morning. As he landed, the pilot radioed that he had only enough fuel to stay on the ground four minutes— get the patient on in a hurry.

Six Sherpas carried the stretcher out of the tent and ran at a trot over the rocky moraine toward the landing area as another Sherpa ran alongside holding the IV. The drama was spectacular. The entire Everest base camp watched as a single person. I ran a little ahead of the stretcher, as did Peter, radio in hand, talking to the pilot. We crossed a frozen pond. The helicopter was only about a hundred yards further on, where a crowd of people were keeping their distance around it. The pilot, afraid he wouldn't be able to start up again if he shut down, kept the blades spinning, sending up a storm of driven snow and ice. I ran ahead through the snow and the crowd and the deafening rotor noise and jumped into the helicopter through the open back door. It was a spare-looking military model, stripped down to be as light as possible. As the Sherpas approached, I folded the backseat down and pointed the end of the stretcher into the door. Grasping it with both hands, I pulled it in while they pushed. It came in faster than I expected and momentarily went half out the other side. Peter handed me the IV and I hung it from a piece of metal protruding from the back wall. A Sherpa threw in Pasang's knapsack and the pilot threw it right back out again. He wasn't going to take any extra weight. And he had already been on the ground more than four minutes. I jumped out and shut the door. Peter yelled at everybody to get away and get down. The pilot revved up the rotors and a snowstorm blew over us for what seemed like a long time but probably was less than a minute. Then with a roar that reverberated through the valley, the helicopter lifted off and disappeared over the mountains.

Suddenly there was silence; and then everyone started talking at once. We could feel the excitement all around us. Peter, Anil, and I shook hands and patted each other on the back repeatedly. We were smiling broadly and had tears in our eyes. We had managed to keep this Sherpa alive through a long day and night. Our job was finished—in two hours he'd be in Kathmandu.

Buoyed by my medical performance I was determined to try the mountain again, so after relaxing the rest of the morning, I set out once more for the icefall. This time I wanted to go alone, feel how my body was doing and set my own pace. If I climb "within myself" I can develop an internal rhythm, shifting gears when necessary to minimize engine wear. Besides all that, if I looked bad, I'd rather be by myself.

A light snow was falling and there was no wind. This passes for a pleasant afternoon on Everest. The first part of the icefall is safe to climb alone because it's at a relatively low angle. A fall would just result in a long, but more or less gentle, slide. I went a lot higher than before, reaching the anchoring screw for the first fixed rope, a green one, which rose steeply around an ice pinnacle and disappeared into the unknown above me. This was a smart place to stop and was actually a very pleasant spot. I took a few minutes to watch a small soundless avalanche high up on the southwest face. Although I felt better in the icefall than I had yesterday, I still had to stop and admire the view a lot more often than I wanted to. I seemed to be a lot better at medicine than mountaineering.

The dinner clang followed by the dreaded cry "soup ready!" came too soon. I waited as long as I could and then came out of my refuge to get the meal over with. The only seat left was in the corner far from the propane heater and next to the frequently opened tent door, so it was cold. Eating with my gloves on, I listened to the latest report on the buildup of supplies. We had fifty loads at Camp I and sixteen at Camp II. We would be able to move up to Camp I tomorrow night. The conversation then changed to a series of increasingly boring climbing adventures followed by stories about people I didn't know. I was cold, the social scene was getting on my nerves, and I couldn't wait to get out of there.

John asked Todd, "So how far is it to the first fixed rope? About a third of the way up the icefall?"

I guessed to myself about a tenth but I wanted to be pessimistic so I could be pleasantly surprised.

Todd replied, "Up to there doesn't even count. The fixed rope is the start."

That wasn't something I wanted to hear. I said good-bye, filling my insulated water bottle with boiling water as I left.

Despite the hot water bottle between my feet that was slowly radiating heat into the sleeping bag, I couldn't warm up. And dinner was an immovable lump in my stomach. At first I was afraid I was going to throw up, but as the sleepless night wore on, I began hoping I would. A strong wave of nausea hit me at some unknown hour in the darkness, and amazingly I was able to find the two zippers to open my tent door quickly. Without coming out of my sleeping bag, I stuck my head out of the tent and threw up. Three times. My head was just an inch above the cold rocks and a pool of moonlit vomit. In twenty-eight hours I was supposed to go up the icefall to Camp I. I hoped this would be the lowest point of the trip.

Sound carries well at night. The whole camp knew I had been sick and with the morning light came visitors with tea, hot soup, candy bars, and amateur medical advice. I had slept with all my clothes on and felt pretty raunchy but it was too cold, or I was too cold, to take a shower. Ong-Chu brought me a basin of steaming hot water, which I left just outside my tent while I stripped down inside and used a rag to wash my critical areas.

Feeling better, and surprisingly clean, I finally made it out of my tent.

"You know, for a good doctor, you're a lousy patient," Todd opined.

He was right. I had allowed myself to get dehydrated yesterday. We were living in a refrigerator: Only the coldest and driest air is light enough to float up to Everest. That inhaled air has to be warmed and moistened before it reaches the lungs, and most of the added moisture is lost when the air is exhaled. The harder you breathe, the more water you lose. I had been telling everybody to drink at least four liters a day but I hadn't taken my own advice.

My muscles had dried out, leaving me weak and tired. My stomach had refused to work, which is why the food made a U-turn last night. With water added I was walking to the New Zealand tent, but not quite ready to try eating.

Their food might be a little more enticing than ours, but that was not why I was going.

A cute girl in a baseball cap offered me tea and cookies, which I accepted and held in both hands. Doctors were milling around holding teacups and making small talk like they do at a cocktail party before a medical convention. Just as I found a comfortable box to sit on the girl in the baseball cap called the meeting to order. She was Jan Arnold, Rob Hall's girlfriend and the New Zealand team doctor. She had just arrived and wanted to thank all of us for our splendid cooperation on behalf of her Sherpa. She had gotten word that he was now conscious and taking fluids. An American doctor who runs a clinic in Kathmandu arranged to have him met at the airport and brought to a first-rate facility. We had been uneasy about the level of care he would get since, in Nepal, as everywhere else in the world including the United States, the quality of medical care can vary enormously depending on social status. Sherpas are at the low end of the spectrum so we were afraid Pasang would be left in a hallway somewhere and were happy to hear that he was doing well. When Jan asked if anyone had anything else to add, Peter said, "Someone's been replacing our titanium screws in the icefall with cheaper aluminum ones. If we find out who it is, we're going to blow his fingers off."

On that note the meeting came to an end with everyone agreeing to meet again next week. I hoped that by then I'd be at Camp I. I'd already been to more medical meetings at base camp than I'd go to in a year in New York.

I wouldn't be going anywhere if I didn't get my gear packed. I still needed to reduce the amount of "essential" stuff I'd be taking up tomorrow. I laid out my equipment and Vern came over to help.

"It looks like you need to do some serious damage to that pile," Vern said. This is a guy who saves weight by using his water bottle as a pee bottle also. By the time we were finished I was wondering why I needed to take anything at all.

Before heading up to Camp I, we had to hold a *puja,* a ceremony to ask for safe passage through the mountain. The Sherpas wouldn't consider climbing without it. Neither would we.

At the highest point in our camp, a neat square stone altar, the lhapso, had been built out of the surrounding rubble. In the center was a tall wooden pole cut from a forested region below and laboriously carried up by two Sherpas—each holding one end. From the top of the pole colorful prayer flags were strung out in various directions, angling down to the surrounding rocks like signal flags on a sailboat. Each expedition had its own lhapso, and the overall effect made base camp look like a carnival.

Cut into the front of the lhapso was a shelf on which juniper branches were stacked. The base of the monument rested on a flat platform lined with offerings of rice, barley, flour, and sweets—in our case Milky Way bars, Reese's peanut butter cups, and M&M's.

Many Sherpas grow up with the idea of becoming lamas, but the discipline is rigorous and some, after attaining the lower level of monkhood, decide that climbing Mount Everest might be easier. Two of these "monks" on our expedition led the service. We sat on the rocks around the lhapso and watched as the juniper branches were lit, creating an intentionally smoky fire. Juniper smoke is holy and, as the wind shifted repeatedly, we could tell by the coughing which part of the crowd was being blessed.

Snow began to fall, obscuring the vast background and intimately enclosing our little ceremony. The chanting took on a hushed tone. Chang was offered all around. Leaning against one side of the lhapso was a collection of ice axes which expedition members had brought out earlier to be included in the blessing. I regretted that I hadn't been around earlier to take mine out but then watched as each ax was smeared with yak butter, including mine. Someone had been thoughtful enough to go to my tent and find my ax while I had been busy elsewhere in the New Zealand tent.

Rice was passed around and at the appropriate moment there was a shout—the cue to throw a handful into the fire. Each of us then was given a tiny bag of rice which was tied onto our red necklaces—this was our lucky rice, to accompany us throughout the expedition and not to be taken off until we were safely down from the mountain.

As the ceremony concluded, the snow got heavier and everyone retreated to their tents. I wasn't yet fully organized to go up the icefall and now, with the snow, I had to work with all my gear cramped inside to make my final adjustments. I was thinking that all the others must be asleep already and that I had so much left to do, when I heard Todd's voice from just outside the tent.

"Hey, Ken, we decided not to go tomorrow. There's too much new snow on the route. I just thought I'd let you know so you could take it easy."

Exactly right. That was great news. An extra day was just what I needed. I relaxed, and then started to think how the snow had begun as the puja got under way, intensifying as the prayers were completed. The thought almost made me uneasy. I was being rewarded for my medical work with an extra day. It was another example of unrelated events having the cosmic connection Josiane and I believed in.

It's a great feeling to wake up in a warm sleeping bag, feel the cold air on your face and realize you don't have to get up. I waited until Everest's huge shadow retreated upvalley past me and the sun warmed my tent.

Extra time leads to extra thinking, particularly one day before a big event. I was sitting on a rock in front of my tent, watching a yak (part of a herd that came to resupply us) eat a cardboard box and wondering if my time wouldn't be better spent at home with my family. I was deep in thought and didn't notice the usually talkative Margo until she sat down next to me. With no preamble, she said, "Every day I ask myself why I'm here."

It was a surprising comment from someone who had climbed big mountains all over the world and seemed very at home at base camp. I told her, "I feel that way every morning, but by the afternoon I feel better. The sun helps."

She liked hearing that. "I'm glad I'm not the only one."

John came up next. "You know, Doc, that partial ligament tear in my knee that I told you about? It was really a complete tear. I didn't tell you because I was afraid what your reaction would be, but I feel better with you knowing."

Suddenly it seemed like we had passed a critical threshold on Everest. The icefall was looming just ahead of us and people were anxious to remove their facades and square their accounts. Facing danger often impels one to remove the superficial layers that impede real contact with other people. It has a cleansing effect on the soul and is one of the abiding attractions of mountaineering.

Todd came to join our little support group and we were eager to hear words of wisdom from our expedition leader: "Wasn't it a beautiful sight at the puja yesterday, to see all those flags blowing in the wind, carrying our prayers? Last year I brought a string of prayer flags home for my mother to hang in her backyard while I was away. She had to take them down though. The civic association in her neighborhood told her she couldn't hang her laundry outside."

So much for abstract philosophy. In my tent that evening, I kept busy rearranging items I might need during the night, like my headlight, tissues and pee bottle, and then settled into my sleeping bag with a few reminders. Tomorrow would be my first big test on Everest. Jonathan thought it would be good if I could hear music on the mountain whenever I wanted to, and now seemed like the right time. I wound up the little music box he had given me and in the silent tent heard the clear metallic tones of "Somewhere over the Rainbow." Jennifer had given me a snow globe, which she thought would be appropriately relaxing for my trip. Shaking the water, it created a tranquil winter scene of gently settling "snow" particles—except that tonight the water was frozen. To carry out her simple-hearted intention, I took the snow globe into my sleeping bag to thaw it out. Last, I took out a picture of Josiane. It was the same picture I always carried but this time she looked especially cute. What did I need to go up the icefall for?

CHAPTER

5

Awakening an hour early, I knew instantly I was too nervous to go back to sleep. In the quiet of the night I savored the warm comfort of my sleeping bag until I heard two Sherpas coming around to each tent loudly whispering "Good morning."

I switched on my headlamp, the first in a series of irrevocable moves leading to the icefall. The snow globe had been inside my sleeping bag all night and, now defrosted, was showing the scene Jennifer had intended for me to see. The pee bottle, lying outside my bed and used twice during the night, was a different story. It was frozen solid. Poking my ice ax through the opening of the bottle, I chopped the urine into chunks small enough to be shaken out. Once empty, the bottle was added to my backpack. My homemade dolls jumped into my chest pocket—three lightweight reminders not to take any chances on the mountain.

Everything up to now had been done from inside the sleeping bag. With all my mountaineering experience, I still haven't found a way to roll up my sleeping bag without getting out of it first. Now I had to take that second irrevocable step. The sleeping bag was rolled and tied and I was now fully packed. Only the third, final step remained: I had to separate from my tent. I opened the zipper and looked out at the black night, pausing like a swimmer about to dive into a pool of cold water.

Most of the tents were lit opaquely from within, looking like lampshades scattered around the camp. There were already some headlights moving about by the mess tent. I didn't want to be the last one out. Simple fear of embarrassment can be a strong motivator, and suddenly I was outside the tent.

When I have a long day in the operating room, I try to do the least enjoyable case first so that I can be relaxed for any difficulties that come later. It applies on the mountain as well, so the job I tried to get rid of first was going to the bathroom. But I wasn't the only one with that idea. From outside my tent I looked down the ravine in the direction of the darkness around the outhouse. There was a solitary stationary light that didn't move for quite a while. Someone was having a tough time there. When the light finally moved away, I started down the ravine, but before I could get very far a second light switched on near the first. Someone had been waiting patiently in the dark and was up next. My turn came soon after, and as I finished, another moving light appeared. It was a silent but orderly dance of fireflies.

I went back to my tent to create some semblance of cleanliness. We would be gone a few days and hygiene would only get tougher higher up. Dropping my pants, I cleaned myself with baby wipes and then put a fresh sanitary napkin in the bottom of my underwear, which I could change daily to keep the underwear from getting too dirty. I smiled at the idea of my climbing companions discovering these things in my tent if I didn't come back and wondering if they had been climbing with a transvestite. As a final precaution I put an extra pair of underwear in my backpack just in case. Using it now would be too extravagant. The pair I had on was only two days old.

The heater was going, the lantern was lit, and food was on the table. The mess tent was an oasis in the darkened camp. I was glad to see not everyone had arrived yet. Climbers were sitting around, not talking much, making last-minute unnecessary adjustments to their equipment. I relaced my boots to make them just a little bit tighter, then did the laces a third time back to the way they were before.

Without a formal word from anyone, it was suddenly time to go and we all got up together. Outside, the fire from the lhapso drew us in like a beacon in the night. Ong-Chu was there to put rice in our hands to throw in the flame and to make sure each of us was blessed by juniper smoke before we started off. So serious was he about his job that he called back one climber who set off before the smoke had been blown over him.

A line of lights, with me in the middle, moved up the moraine. Loose rocks and stiff climbing boots don't make a good match. My knee was already complaining from the effort of accommodating to the uneven terrain. By the time I reached the crampon point, most of the good sitting rocks were taken but I found a small pointy one I could rest on to gear up and catch my breath (already).

From out of my backpack came all my hardware: helmet, harness, and two crampons which I dropped in front of me on a flat spot in the ice. Crampons are adjustable metal platforms that fit on the bottoms of rigid-soled boots with ten triangular spikes projecting downward and two more projecting forward. Each crampon closed snugly around my boot as I stepped into it, locking in place with a reassuring snap.

Next was the harness: a web of nylon straps placed over my butt, brought forward around my hips and up through my crotch, cinched together tightly enough in front so that I wouldn't fall out even if I were hanging upside down. Tightening the strap between my legs must be done just so, otherwise being suspended right side up could prove a lot more painful than being upside down.

The most annoying piece of equipment is the helmet. The only place we wear it is in the icefall, where the risk of tumbling into a crevasse or getting bopped with falling ice outweighs the annoyance. It seemed especially confining now, with the tight chin strap making it hard for me to swallow. With our headlights fastened to the front of our helmets, still in the dark, we looked like miners about to descend into the mountain rather than climbers about to move over it.

The Khumbu Icefall is part of the legend. Every account of Everest from the south side talks about it. We were about to climb a slow-motion waterfall—the source of the flow being the snow and ice on the flanks of three mountains: Everest, Lhotse, and Nuptse. They funnel together into the frozen river of the Western Cwm Glacier, spilling abruptly over the edge at the top of the icefall, two thousand vertical feet above where we stood right now. This was the gateway to the upper reaches of Everest—the route that allowed it to be climbed for the first time. It was a dangerous pathway through a jumble of seracs (ice blocks the size of buildings) and over crevasses (cracks in the ice that run ten stories deep). All of it was on the move, subjected to daily heating from the sun and relentless pressure from the ice above. Sudden fractures in the ice cause the seracs to topple without warning and the crevasses to open or close overnight. Surveying this turbulent scene for the first time, Sir

Edmund Hillary said, "Everest can be climbed by this route, but we have to raise the level of acceptable risk."

Was I taking an acceptable risk? How can any risk be acceptable if it's unnecessary? But I had thought this through many times and now was not the time for misgivings. Distraction could be deadly. I lost myself in the imperatives of the climb.

The circle of snow illuminated by my headlamp was all I could see of the majestic icefall. Though mindful of the extraordinary day which was beginning now, I was nevertheless concentrating only on the steps I was taking, setting a pace to keep my breathing under control. Within my little spotlight I listened to the rhythmic clanking of my carabiners hitting against each other and felt the familiar repeated crunch of my crampons compressing the snow beneath my feet.

The route started by twisting and swirling around "little" snow mounds that were far taller than I. I had entered a maze—openings in every direction bordered by walls I couldn't see over. With each climber moving at his own pace, we quickly were spread out enough to lose sight of each other around the repeated turns. I was dependent for direction on following the trail of compacted snow created over days by previous climbers. Yesterday's snowfall, however, had dusted the trail in many places, reducing me to searching for fresh crampon prints to follow. I was glad to have a narrowly focused activity that literally made me concentrate on moving one step at a time in the right direction. At this early point, if I fully realized where I was and what I was trying to do, it might be too daunting and defeating.

At any moment I expected to see the first fixed line—the green rope where I had turned around on my daylight practice run. The trail coursed up and down and around, but mostly up. It gradually occurred to me that we were taking a different route since we would otherwise have passed that rope already. I realized I must be well into the icefall by now, moving more efficiently than I thought, keeping my feet in balance and my breathing under control. Emboldened by my progress, I looked up to scan the ice around me and caught a glimpse of a black rope anchored up ahead. The slope wasn't steep and, feeling strong, I increased my pace to reach it. The additional light as I approached showed the "black" rope to be green, and with a sinking feeling I understood that only now was I getting to the beginning of the icefall.

Deflated by my mental setback and by the little burst of speed that had put me outside my steady rhythm, I paused at the anchor to catch my breath. This had been the rope that I thought "rose around an ice pinnacle and disappeared into the unknown" when I had stood here in the daylight two days ago. Once I stopped panting, I grabbed the rope for balance, kicked my feet into the slope, and grunted my way up and over this first obstacle. There was nothing poetic about it now.

By the increasing angle of the icefall I knew I was progressing from the lower spill-out zone to the vertical midsection where the ice falls more rapidly and chaotically. Increased turbulence means more instability and more danger but it also creates bizarre and beautiful ice forms. I was surrounded by improbable ice sculptures, from delicate carvings to fluted spires and sheer walls towering hundreds of feet over me. Caught momentarily in my headlight, the exquisite shapes were alluring, inviting me to rest and admire them like the call of a siren's song, but lingering too long in this part of the icefall could prove deadly.

Ahead of me I could see two climbers' lights. They weren't far away but they were way high above me so I knew a steep section was coming up. A third light appeared, brighter, still higher, and directly above the other two. But it wasn't a headlight, it was moonrise over the icefall. I shut off my headlight. Suddenly there was a silver glow on all the seracs and slopes and formations. I was climbing in fantasyland.

Crevasses riddled the ice and a large one loomed ahead. We had already crossed a few small ones by "simply" jumping over them though no jump is simple when you are carrying a twenty-pound pack, wearing three layers of pants, and shoes that weigh four pounds each.

The chasm was twenty feet across and ten stories deep. An aluminum ladder was laid across it, anchored tightly at each end by ropes tied to ice screws. Two additional slack ropes spanned the chasm, one along either side of the ladder, held independently by another set of ice screws. Climbers tend to collect at these ladders since only one person can be on at a time and because crossing is a little easier if someone else is there to help with the ropes.

"Looking good, Ken," John said as I approached. It gave me a little lift to hear him say it, even though I knew it wasn't so. After a few deep breaths I was about to respond but then, as if to prove he was wrong, the cold air deep in my lungs set off a fit of coughing. I finished by blowing my nose and didn't say anything.

John got on the ladder and I stepped up behind him to the edge of the crevasse, grabbing both slack ropes and leaning backward to create enough tension so the ropes would rise to his waist level. John clipped in to both of these safety ropes so that if he fell off the ladder, he'd still be suspended by the ropes. By bringing the ropes up to his arms I was allowing him to also use them as railings for balance. Once across, he unclipped and said, "Thanks," signaling to me that I could relax the ropes and that he wouldn't be falling in.

Frank came up behind me to hold the ropes and to remark, "You know, back home in Hong Kong, if you laid a ladder between the roofs of two ten-story buildings and told me to walk across, I'd say you were crazy."

With that thought I clipped in and started across the crevasse. The trick to getting to the other side is to find a position in which your spiked boot will fit securely onto rungs that have a lot of space between them. Everyone's crampons are different so everyone has to find his own technique. My secret was to have a foot big enough to span two rungs, placing my back-most point behind one rung and my front points over the next at the same time. The system worked well except that I had to remember to lift my toe before my heel for each step—an awkward but necessary maneuver, otherwise my front points would curl around the rung and pin me to the ladder.

Successfully crossing the crevasse entitled all of us to cross more crevasses and we soon lost track of the number. The moon completed its narrow arc from the southwest shoulder of Everest to the ridge of Nuptse, over which it disappeared. Soft predawn light illuminated first the pinnacles and ice walls and later the bottoms of even the deepest crevasses.

"So this is what we've been doing all night," John said as he stood in the middle of a ladder, looking between his feet at the hard blue ice far below. "If I had seen this before, I would have headed back to my tent. No wonder we start in the dark."

Frozen blood streaked the wall of one crevasse and left a small red stain at the bottom, a jarring reminder of reality to those of us who had been lulled by the abstract beauty around and below us. This was where the Sherpa had stumbled on the ladder and fallen in. He hadn't bothered to clip in because the crossing was too easy.

The cold was more penetrating now, as it always is just before dawn. We were in the "popcorn" section—a collection of crumbly looking ice blocks set at a steep angle and about ready to topple over. The route worked its way through them, more vertical than before, forcing me to chop holes in the ice with my ax so I could move up using my hands and feet together. Exhausting work, but I seemed to be getting more exhausted than anyone else.

I had been climbing with Skip, who had been slowing his pace to stay with me, but as we came under a particularly ominous overhang and I started to lag behind, Skip said, "I'll move on ahead and wait for you at the other end."

I said, "Sure, no point in this thing falling on both of us," but what I thought was, What do you think I'm going to do here, stop for a picnic? I was angry at myself for not being able to move faster and felt abandoned. He was right, of course. In the end everyone climbs Everest by himself.

Just beyond the popcorn the sun rose. The ice opened out into a little field where there were no towering walls to threaten us or to block the sunshine. Skip, John, and a few others were sitting on their packs, eating and relaxing. I was anxious to get out of the shadows and join them. I needed to rest, warm up, and feel that I had caught up.

As I was making myself comfortable, the party was suddenly over and everyone else moved on. I stripped off some layers of clothes that sunrise had made excessive and put on sunblock, lip balm, and sunglasses. Taking out my water bottle and a chocolate bar, I dined alone.

Pete popped out of the popcorn. I was glad to see him but he was the sweeper—the strongest climber, staying intentionally last to be sure no one was left behind. He confirmed that everyone had passed me.

"How much further ahead are the others?" Pete asked.

"They left just as I got here. I'm trying not to take it personally."

With the sun up, ice blocks would be starting to melt and we still had to cross the bowling alley—a narrow up-ramp with no place to hide on either side if a frozen ball came tumbling down looking for a strike.

Pete, in his usual understated way, said, "Perhaps you'd like to move through here a little more rapidly." I responded to the gentle tug on my invisible reins and increased my speed—not nearly as fast as Pete could have gone if he were alone, but he stayed with me and we got through without any points being scored.

We were nearing the top of the icefall now and like any waterfall, the flow is smoother and rounder where it starts. The angle lessened and the crevasses became larger and more orderly, forming long parallel rows. To span some of the crevasses several ladders were tied together end to end with climbing rope. One of the last was a tenuous four-ladder construction which bent inexorably downward as my weight moved across it until at the halfway point I was unable to see over either rim. With the oscillation from each step I was bobbing close enough to the bottom to see the sprinkled holy rice cast into the crevasse by Sherpas who had suddenly been inspired to ask for an additional blessing. It seemed like a good idea to me, too.

Finally the crevasses became too wide. The only way to cross was to down-climb into them on the near side and climb back out on the far side. The back wall of the last big crevasse rose up to form a near-vertical serac—the final obstacle of the icefall. Three ladders were set on the lower part of the wall but they had frozen against the ice, forcing us to climb with only room enough for toe holds on each rung. Above the top ladder was a fixed rope with which I hauled myself up, finding footholds as I went but resting between each step. I climbed past the ragged remnant of a tent embedded in the ice. It had been left behind at Camp I last year and was slowly flowing down the icefall. It couldn't have gone too far in one year, I reasoned optimistically. I must be close to the camp.

The angle lessened again and the climbing got easier. The fixed rope ended at a flat spot where a sheet of aluminum was sticking up out of the ice. On it, someone had scrawled, "Welcome to the Western Cwm."

I sat down next to it to catch my breath and wait for Pete, who couldn't start up the last rope until I was off it. I noticed Todd watching me from a higher ridge. He gave me the thumbs-up sign and I returned it. Pete came up, and out of consideration for me, remarked how tough that last part of the climb was, but he didn't even have the decency to be out of breath when he said it.

The remaining way to our camp wasn't very long or very steep but it seemed to be both. I was very tired. Up ahead I could see the camp and, to my surprise, some climbers were just now arriving. I wasn't so far behind and after one last annoying rise that seemed like another mountain, I was there.

Camp I was four tents huddled close together and tightly enclosed by a round wall of ice blocks that looked like an open-air igloo. Built on the first flat spot our advance party of Sherpas could find, it sat like a fort on a small plateau just upstream from the edge of the icefall.

I was greeted by the sounds of heavy breathing mixed with repetitive nose blowing and dry hacking coughs—a high altitude cacophony created by prolonged strenuous exertion in cold dry air and a relatively sudden elevation gain of two thousand feet. Most of the orchestra members were sitting on their packs outside the ice wall, the camp being too small to sit within. A few others were already inside, showing signs of life either by arranging their tents or moaning. I immediately identified with those on the outside, and sat down to do a little breathing and enjoy the sun. After five hours in the icefall it was hard to believe it was still early in the morning.

As Vern and Skip were melting snow to make tea, Skip recounted the excitement he felt climbing through the famous Khumbu Icefall; it was one of the biggest thrills of his climbing career. True enough, the place is legendary and that was part of the reason we were all here, but for the moment I was finding it hard to think in those lofty abstractions. I'd save that for later.

The tea tasted great. Fluids, plus some rest and sunshine, were bringing me back to life but apparently more slowly than the others. John was already sawing ice blocks to add to our wall, while Hugh was out prospecting with a shovel, looking for firmer snow that would give a greater quantity of water when melted. Ever-thoughtful Frank was working on accommodations, assigning John and myself to his tent, then inflating our air mattresses (no mean trick in the thin air at 19,500 feet) and rolling out our sleeping bags. He was a regular hotelier.

I needed to walk so I could move more air through my lungs. Todd volunteered to walk with me. We stayed on the uphill side of the plateau so that if we slipped on the slick ice we would slide into the camp and not over the edge of the icefall.

"You know, it's funny," Todd said. "Everyone here is an experienced mountaineer but when they get on Everest they forget everything and start asking dumb questions like what kind of socks to bring to Camp One."

We were walking at the bottom of the Western Cwm—a glacier that rose another two thousand feet above us. On the right was Nuptse and ahead was Lhotse. The enormous peak of Everest was still out of sight behind the west ridge and lost in the clouds.

"I know what you mean," I answered. "But I also understand how Everest is so daunting, it can have that effect on people."

We watched clouds form far below and then slowly rise up the valley toward us. They reached the top of the icefall and we were enveloped in fog. The clouds had arrived at Camp I.

Seeking refuge from the cold damp air, I joined John and Frank in our two-man tent. Being the last one in, the only spot left was between the others—sort of like the middle airplane seat on an economy flight, but at least it would be warmed by bodies on either side.

Vern's arm appeared through our tent door, his open hand signaling that he was ready to take our mugs. One by one he filled them with the pea soup he had just heated. He could reach into every tent just by turning around from his spot outside next to the cook stove. The camp was so small there was no need for him to get up.

Next Vern read out the labels on the frozen food packets: "Okay, who wants beef stew, who wants fiesta chicken, and who wants ravioli?"

Frank was in a quandary. "It depends . . . are you serving red or white wine?"

My order of ravioli was ready before I was, and it got dumped into my mug still half-filled with pea soup. Frank got stew instead of chicken and loudly protested that he wanted to see the chef.

"Listen Frank," Vern reasoned, "it doesn't matter. All the packets taste the same anyway."

The only way to empty my mug without getting out of the tent was to eat its contents, but I had no appetite, especially for soggy ravioli. I was too tired and too warm to get out and dump it so I put it aside and dully settled back in my sleeping bag. With my eyes closed I listened to camp noises that gradually seemed to grow more and more distant.

Vern was on the radio to base camp. Dimly, I listened to the sound of his voice but not the words, until the phrase "sounds like a bad burn" penetrated my ears. I waited on the brink of consciousness for the next few critical seconds. Either I'd hear my name or else I could go back to my stupor.

"Uh, Ken," Vern called from outside the tent, "we've got a Sherpa who needs some help." Instantly awake, I came out of the tent and took the radio Vern offered up to me.

Sonang, one of our porters, had been carrying a leaky kerosene container in his pack and now the skin on his back was red, blistered, and painful. It was a second-degree chemical burn. I advised Liz to apply burn cream and not to break the blisters or let him carry anything that might break them—steps that would ease his pain and help prevent infection. And lastly, an instruction that would probably be the hardest to carry out: "Try to find him a clean shirt."

I was now too tired to fall asleep. Laid out like stacked logs, we had no room in the tent to turn around nor even enough space for me to bend my knees up—a near requirement for me to sleep. I hadn't had the forethought to throw out my ravioli when I left the tent but I was glad I remembered to take a pee before I got back inside—using the pee bottle in here would be risky, if I could go at all.

Every three minutes it seemed like Frank died. In his sleep, his rapid, shallow breathing was followed by a long period—thirty seconds or more—of no breathing at all, then the cycle would resume. This was the Cheyne-Stokes phenomenon, very common at altitude. The body depends on a buildup of carbon dioxide to stimulate respiration but in thin air short, frequent breaths keep its concentration in the blood too low. Lungs forget to breathe until the gas slowly reaccumulates and gets them going again. Interesting to read about but unnerving to listen to.

I guess I finally fell asleep because suddenly it was light out. I awoke to the sound of Vern cleaning the dishes with his ice ax. He was chipping frozen pea soup out of a pot.

One by one we trickled out of our tents. Today would be a rest day. We needed time to adapt to the altitude since a sudden two-thousand-foot gain could play havoc with our bodies.

"Geez, I hope I don't look as bad as you," John said to me by way of greeting.

I could feel I had facial edema—swelling of the face due to accumulation of fluid in the skin—another unpleasant effect of altitude. Also, I didn't remember when I had shaved last and I never comb my hair. Without a mirror I could only speculate on the combined effect.

As I drank a mug full of fresh hot chocolate, mixed with the ravioli left over in my cup from last night, I took a medical survey. Frank's breathing had stabilized. One climber had thrown up during the night and still looked a little queasy this morning. Everyone was tired and several people complained of headaches, nausea, and fatigue. At this altitude these can be early warning signs of pulmonary or cerebral edema, both potentially fatal. The only really effective treatment is immediate rapid descent. The trouble is, the same signs can be due to an upset stomach, dehydration, or just the difficult climb through the icefall yesterday. If I sent down everyone who had a problem, no one would ever climb anything.

It was time to start sorting things out. To those who wanted them, I gave out mild headache pills. Stronger painkillers might mask symptoms too effectively. Everyone was encouraged to drink and eat. No one needed encouragement to rest. In a few hours we'd have a better idea of who had what.

The climber who had thrown up was sitting against the ice wall breathing through his mouth, his head cocked to one side. I sat down next to him.

"Not feeling so good, huh?"

"I think there was too much fiesta in my chicken last night, Doc."

Could be. Too much fiesta chicken can cause vomiting just as surely as cerebral edema can but one can be cured with Pepto-Bismol, while delay in treating the other is fatal. He had a rapid pulse and clammy skin. He looked sick.

I wanted to get him out of there as soon as possible, so I assigned a Sherpa to escort him down. With the drop in altitude as well as some Pepto-Bismol, he would probably get better. If he didn't, the other doctors in base camp could help him out.

Pete came by to find out first about our sick climber and second to ask for ophthalmic solution. He had forgotten to take out his contact lenses last night and now they were fogged over and stuck in his eyes. I had just the thing for it and solved the problem quickly.

"Seeing better now?" I asked, expecting a thank-you as Pete tested his eyes by blinking and looking right at me.

"Yeah, too well," Pete said. "It's scary what our doctor looks like."

No one felt like moving but everyone knew it was no time to be lethargic. Inactivity would gradually close the lungs down by creating a downward spiral in which decreased breathing brought in less oxygen, leading to more fatigue and even less breathing. Exercise would force open extra air sacs that are closed during quiet respiration, adding more channels for airflow to compensate for the lower oxygen content. At this altitude exercise is still effective but as the air thins it takes more and more work to get less and less oxygen. The more efficient your muscles are, the higher you can go before the balance shifts and the amount of air taken in becomes less than what is used up in the effort to get it.

Dutifully, I embarked with the others on a two-hour roundtrip glacier hike. Breathing deeply to put forth the necessary effort, I felt like my balance had shifted already. By the time we returned to Camp I, I felt more acclimatized but, as I took off my crampons and sagged against the ice wall, I wondered if lethargy might not be a better alternative.

Camp I was a stark place right now: a narrow plateau of ice surrounded by crevasses and brightly illuminated by the midday sun. As I was peeling my freshly boiled potatoes with a spoon, I put in a call to base camp and learned that Sonang's blisters were healing and that our vomiting climber was feeling much better. I'll never know if it was the two-thousand-foot descent or the Pepto-Bismol.

A second night at Camp I was approaching and everything seemed to be under control. Tomorrow we would move up to Camp II. Everyone seemed fit and ready to go. I relaxed in my tent and took the luxury of carefully brushing my teeth. Not having a convenient receptacle to spit into, I swallowed the mixture of toothpaste, water, and food particles each time, reasoning that the extra fluid and nutrition would be good for me.

Blue and white were the only colors needed to paint the scene. There was only sky and ice around us, brightly lit by a sun that wasn't even up yet. Our little encampment seemed ridiculously puny amid the overwhelming grandeur of the Western Cwm but it was our haven, and our lives depended on it. In preparation to leave, we collapsed the tents and shoveled some snow on top so that the wind wouldn't be able to reinflate them and blow them over the icefall while we were gone.

The cook tent was the last one to take down. Its high triangular roof made it the most vulnerable to the wind but we couldn't close it until we finished boiling enough water to fill our bottles and to make instant oatmeal for breakfast. Water will not boil if you look at it—it's a basic law of camping—so all of us busied ourselves packing supplies to carry up to Camp II while I made sure we were leaving some essentials behind in the snow: a cache of food and fuel, oxygen tank and regulator, sleeping bag, and stove. Though the plan was to bypass this camp on our way back (descending directly from II to base), we might need a first aid station in an emergency.

Despite occasional glances from all of us, the water finally did boil and oatmeal was served. Frank was the only one who liked it. As his doctor, I had to worry about the state of his health. In the hospital, patients who don't complain about the food are usually pretty sick.

A footstep is depressingly small when taken in the vast Western Cwm. I had gotten exhausted just putting my crampons on and now, with my first steps, I was trying to establish a rhythm that would allow me to catch my breath and still move forward. It wouldn't help to contemplate the towering dimensions around me. I concentrated instead on moving through the section immediately ahead. There was a natural snow bridge spanning the first crevasse and Frank was approaching it. Since these bridges can collapse at any time, a safety line had been strung across it but the anchored end was half buried by a recent snowfall. Frank caught his crampon on it and tripped in the snow. Even though he got up immediately he would need a good rest before he would be ready to clip in and cross the snow bridge. That simple error had left him exhausted.

He smiled as I passed him but his labored breathing was louder than mine and I empathized with him. Empathy on my part wasn't necessary, however, since midway through that same snow bridge my foot broke through and I sank in up to my thigh. I was the third person across and the first two were both heavier than I, but for some reason known only to the snowbridge, it decided to give way at that moment. It didn't collapse; it just left me out of breath with one foot dangling in space through a hole in the bottom.

Oblivious to the majesty around me, I watched the back of Vern's boots as he set the pace and I followed. As in the icefall, contemplating the enormity of the Cwm this early on would be anxiety provoking and therefore energy draining. Much better to wear blinders and keep my focus narrow: My goal for the day was to keep constant the distance between Vern's feet and mine. That would bring me to Camp II.

It was getting hot. I took off a layer of clothes and switched from my wool hat to my wide-brimmed sun hat. One crevasse later, it was gone as I leaned forward to check my footing on a ladder and the hat wafted off my head. I watched it float slowly down into the crevasse. It took a long time to hit the bottom.

Crossing a crevasse is like swimming in water over your head. Once it reaches a certain depth, it doesn't matter how much deeper it gets. Going around the crevasse is different—the longer it is, the longer the detour. Faced with a particularly long one, precisely perpendicular to our route, we were forced to make a traverse to the right, toward Nuptse. I hadn't seen Vern for a while and was beginning to think I was falling far behind, though the others after me didn't seem to be getting any closer. Coming up a slope I was relieved to spot Vern not more than thirty yards to my left. So I wasn't slowing down after all, even though I was getting increasingly hot and tired. As I reached the top of the slope, the space between us opened out and I saw to my dismay that we were separated by the crevasse. Vern was only thirty yards away but to get to where he was I still had several hundred yards of crevasse to go around. Suddenly I was very hot and very tired.

The traverse had brought us right under the flank of Nuptse. It was time to regroup. Nuptse has an annoying habit of avalanching—we'd have to move through here rapidly. We spread out about twenty feet apart, spaced so that an avalanche would only catch one or two of us and the ones who weren't covered could look for the ones who were.

Although fear is a powerful motivator, in the abstract it doesn't overcome fatigue. I didn't have the strength to move rapidly, but if I had seen even one errant snowflake coming off the mountain I'm sure my strength would have returned.

The crevasses got longer and wider until they were too long to walk around and too wide to cross over on ladders. At the edge of one yawning chasm, I "prebreathed" to accumulate some extra oxygen, then turned around, stepped over the edge, and down-climbed, breaking loose a lot of snow as I went. At the bottom of the crevasse, I looked up at the sharply edged circle of blue sky as loose powdery snow gently cascaded down on me. I felt like I was inside the snow globe Jennifer had given me; it was as tranquil as she said it would be.

A transcendent moment to enjoy but nevertheless not a time to forget I was in the bottom of a crevasse. I took hold of the fixed rope dangling down the far wall, clipped in, and made my way up the other side. Remembering to breathe as I kicked my crampons into the wall one step at a time, I paced myself and soon my head was above the rim. I allowed myself to relax. One more step and I'd be over the top but as I lifted my knee, the rope held me back. I had come up on the wrong side of a bollard (an ice bulge) and the rope didn't have enough slack to go around it. I tried to flip the rope over the top to my side of the bulge but it was frozen against the ice. I would have to back down to the bollard and unstick it. Or, I could detach myself from the rope and make the last move to the top without a safety line. It was an easy move and it would save a lot of energy. I opted to go down and unstick the rope. We'd already seen how unprotected "easy" moves led to crevasses with red streaks.

That last move sapped my energy—all the more because it was unanticipated and came after I had already started to relax. I was glad to see Vern a few steps behind the rim sitting on his pack and eating. He was well installed and looked like he had been waiting a long time for a bus.

"Would you like some oysters or truffles?" he asked as I approached.

"Wait a minute, are you the same guy who drinks out of his pee bottle?"

I wasn't sure until I saw him spread jelly on the oysters and then actually eat them. That was more like the Vern I knew.

I reached into my pack for a snack and came out with a handful of brown goop. My chocolate bar had melted all over the top compartment, creating a chocolate-covered compass and a chocolate-covered Swiss Army knife.

"Yeah, it's really hot today," Vern said as he surveyed my mess and then downed another oyster.

The Cwm was becoming incredibly hot. Through a thinned-out atmosphere the sun reflected off the snowy slopes of Nuptse, Lhotse, and Everest, concentrating its ultraviolet rays on us like a huge sun reflector at the beach.

While I was deciding whether to drink my liter of water or use it to wash my hand, Skip, Frank, John, Hugh, and Mike arrived, all sweating profusely. Mike had a little thermometer dangling from his pack which read 97 degrees. Heat exhaustion and sunburn were now imminent dangers—all the more so because the idea of heat stroke on Mount Everest is so incongruous.

There was never a real temptation to wash my hand since heat exhaustion is best prevented by adequate fluid intake. I simply wiped my hand on the ice and like the others, downed a liter of water. I reminded everyone to apply sunblock to every part of exposed skin. The intense ultraviolet radiation in the Cwm is reflected at all angles, including straight up, so it's capable of causing burns on eyelids, under chins, and even inside nostrils. Our last precaution was to strip down to a single layer of polypropylene before we started off again. Sustained exertion could cause dangerous heat buildup, so we'd finish the climb in our long underwear.

Margo and Pete came up over the rim as we were packing away our excess clothing. It must have been a strange sight.

Margo asked, "Did we miss something?"

Mike replied, "No, you're just in time. There's no point in a bunch of guys taking their clothes off if there are no women around."

Camp II was bobbing in and out of sight like a buoy far off in the ocean. The angle of the Cwm was more gradual now, so the flow of the glacier was less tumultuous and there were no more crevasses. The terrain was an endless series of ice mounds—frozen waves. The cluster of multicolored specks that was Camp II rhythmically appeared as we mounted the crest of each wave and then disappeared as we descended into the trough.

Slowly the tent colors seemed to get brighter, but the tents never seemed to get closer. The group gradually spread out until each of us was climbing alone, absorbed in his own thoughts, crossing an ocean of ice.

A figure far behind me caught my eye. Though it was a barely discernible speck, I knew it was a Sherpa by the way he moved. Sherpas have a light-stepping, almost jaunty gait that tells you right away they are at home in the mountains.

At each crest I saw the figure drawing closer and, discouragingly quickly, he caught up to me. I didn't recognize him but he smiled, said hello, and passed on by. He disappeared over the next ice wave and reappeared at the crest of another but then he was out of sight completely. Everything was again as it had been and I was alone on a quiet frozen sea. I began to wonder if he had been here at all or if I had just imagined him.

Progress was slow and the route was endless but there was no thought of stopping, much less of turning around. In my mind I removed those options. I no longer had control of the train I was on and it wouldn't stop until it reached its destination. I was suffering and my rhythm was pathetic, but I was on autopilot and my body was proceeding without me.

A black smudge between the glacier and the southwest slope of Everest slowly expanded and became recognizable as a lateral moraine—a deposit of ground-up gravel and boulders scoured out by the friction of ice on rock. This was the place we put Camp II since rock is more stable and warmer than ice, but it was approachable only by a steep and icy slope. Reluctantly I climbed that final obstacle to Camp II.

The first flat rock was really comfortable. As I was thinking about getting my crampons off, Dawa came out of the cook tent with the best slice of canned pineapple I ever ate. I was sitting at the bottom of a gravel chute made into a camp by placing tents, one above the other, on leveled-out steps all the way up the slope. It looked like a residential street in San Francisco.

Vapor rose from my underwear as the sun slowly burned off five hours of accumulated sweat. Climbers straggled in one by one and took positions nearby. None of us talked much. We were all recharging our batteries, resting like reptiles on hot rocks.

John was by far the last to arrive, looking like he had been through a war. Crawling onto a rock next to mine, he was even more discouraged when he realized he was the last reptile. At thirty-one, he was the youngest member of the team and I had just the medical fact he needed.

"The younger you are, the longer it takes to acclimatize," I mentioned casually.

"Really? Really?" His face brightened and I could see a little more energy returning to his body.

The sun lasted just long enough to dry my underwear. As soon as the sky clouded over, it became too cold to sit out and I reluctantly started up the gravel slope to my tent. A crevasse ran transversely through the camp about halfway up. It was narrow enough to step over but just a little too wide to be safe to do it repeatedly. The Sherpas had dumped in enough gravel in one spot to make a bridge across it, marking off the rest of the crevasse with red warning wands. Once across safely, I staggered into my tent and collapsed.

The music of Mozart from Frank's cassette player filled the air as he went about setting up our tent. My other roommate, John, was a semicomatose blob in the corner. The three of us were often together, since Frank felt I was pretty refined for an American and he considered John to be a "diamond in the rough" who lacked exposure to the finer things. I had no desire to help, but the longer I watched

Frank the more I felt obligated to do something. I was saved just in time.

"Frank," John said, without even opening his eyes, "will you stop moving around and turn that crap off so I can sleep?"

Either because of lucky physiology or else because I'm so tired after each day's climb, I sleep soundly in the mountains—except when others can't. That night I dreamed I was alternating between my sleeping bag in Camp II and my bed at home. Where I would be in the morning would be determined by which location my dream was in at the time I awoke.

It was Camp II. John woke me up in the middle of the night to look at Frank, who was having trouble catching his breath. I listened to his lungs: he didn't have pulmonary edema but he wasn't moving a lot of air. He looked scared and that made John scared.

Frank's breath was the only noise we heard—intensified by our closeness within the tent. I gave Frank fluids and diamox—a diuretic with the useful side effect of stimulating breathing—and started a casual conversation with John to lessen the tension and help Frank relax. A long hour later Frank was breathing easier and so were we. John even offered to let Frank put his funky music back on.

In another hour it was sunup, but neither Frank nor I felt like getting out of the tent. John volunteered to bring us breakfast but a few minutes later he was back empty-handed.

"No breakfast in the tents. Todd says everyone's got to get out and move around. You can't stay here if you want oatmeal."

"I'll stay here, then," I said, thinking how tired I was and remembering how tasteless the oatmeal was.

It was seductively comfortable in the tent. I was warm here and had no desire to eat anyway, but moderate activity is important to facilitate acclimatization and the doctor has to set an example. It would be a sensuous pleasure to stay in my sleeping bag but satisfaction comes with not giving in to the easy choices, whether it's getting out of your tent or refusing to quit when you're exhausted.

Tougher choices aren't always smarter choices, and by late morning I was wondering just how smart mountaineers are—a reasonable question to ask myself when I was out above Camp II trying to complete an acclimatization hike despite a freezing wind and wondering where the Cwm was that I climbed yesterday in my underwear. With each step I had to dig in my ski pole on the downwind side to not get blown off course. My face was stinging and my fingers were numb. Leaving my tent had made sense that morning but somehow I couldn't recall the logic right then.

The easy choice can sometimes be the smart choice. I cut my hike short and headed directly for my sleeping bag. When I got to the tent, John was already back, combing ice out of his beard.

"Enjoy your walk, Doc?"

"Yeah, my favorite part was when my hands got so numb I couldn't feel the ski poles."

"For me, it was learning that icicles can hang from nose hairs."

Frank hadn't left the tent since breakfast and was fresh-faced, having spent the morning shaving. He's the only person I know who shaves at Camp II.

"Come on, Frank," John reasoned. "Go for a walk. You don't have to worry about icicles in your beard."

"No thanks, breathing is enough exercise for me today."

The cold was penetrating. My sleeping bag wasn't enough to stop my shaking or slow my respiration. On top of that I had a high-altitude toothache. When there is reduced atmospheric pressure, air that may have gotten trapped between a tooth and its filling expands against a nerve—another delightful mountaineering phenomenon.

It could be worse. One of us could have high altitude flatus. Just as low pressure causes air in teeth to expand, it can cause air in the intestines to expand. The resulting stomach pains can only be relieved by passing gas. You don't have to be a doctor to make the diagnosis. You don't even have to be in the same tent. Out our little window I could see a tent flap opening periodically, followed by the momentary protrusion of an underwear-clad behind. The victim was showing compassion for his tentmates but they must be having a rough time in there.

Twelve hours of interrupted sleep was not enough. My cold throat woke me up repeatedly because I couldn't get my scarf right. The idea was to create an air pocket in front of my mouth—a sort of rebreather that would collect warm, moist air as I exhaled—but the scarf was either wrapped so tightly I couldn't breathe or so loosely the cold air came in "untreated," provoking chills and coughing. By morning, the liner of my sleeping bag was saturated with saliva and I was still tired.

Today we were supposed to hike to the base of Lhotse but no one looked as if he could make it out of the kitchen tent. Swollen faces were everywhere and except for the coughing, there was very little unnecessary motion. I thought I might feel better after breakfast but lost all hope when I saw Dawa serving up corned beef hash mixed with porridge. Incredibly, everyone ate it, then I watched in total disbelief as Frank had seconds. Although I had no appetite at all, Frank somehow cajoled me into finishing a whole bowl.

Later that day on the ice, creeping toward Lhotse, I began to feel betrayed. At breakfast everyone was apparently dead. No one had been able to put both crampons on without resting in between. When we started out it looked like a turtle race, but now everyone was pulling away. John and Frank passed me moving pathetically slowly. In my dimwitted condition it didn't occur to me right away that if they were passing me I must be moving even slower. I felt like shouting, "Wait a minute, we were all supposed to be exhausted together."

The route from above the moraine to the base of Lhotse started with a gradual uphill slope. From near the bottom I watched as, one by one, each turtle disappeared over the top. There was no one in my sight now and no one could see me. Somehow this seemed like an opportunity for me to go even slower since no one would notice—an idea which, unless your brain is low on oxygen, makes no sense at all.

The sun came out and I stopped to remove my jacket and balaclava, but by the time I got them off and into my pack the sky clouded over and I had to take them out again. As I finished putting them on, Frank reappeared at the top of the rise, heading down toward me. I thought he had wiped out and was returning to camp but no, he was coming back to help me, a gesture of true friendship. But that meant he thought I needed help and reluctantly I admitted to myself that I would have felt better if he had come back because he was too tired to go on.

With my escort I made it to the top of the slope, but I felt more and more like a four-cylinder car with only one piston going. Ahead of me were the broad flats, separated from the base of Lhotse by a huge canyon of a crevasse—an obstacle that could only be circumvented by a painfully long detour almost to the edge of Nuptse. At the far side rose an enormous ice ramp running half the length of Lhotse's base, the top blending into the sheer south wall. From there the climb took off in earnest: five thousand more feet of slick ice at an unrelenting forty-five-degree angle. The slope was nearly featureless, but soon an advance party of Sherpas and lead climbers would cut out a notch halfway up, anchor some tents there, and call it Camp III. We would have to get from Camp II to Camp III in a single day. This was the only place on the route where you could see all the way from one camp to another—the distances were just not human size.

The view was overpowering and literally took my breath away, what little of it I had. The ethereal top of Lhotse was obscured by an irregular band of clouds, but beyond and higher still, rising out of those clouds was a dark triangle of rock—the summit of Everest.

I stood still at the top of the rise, feeling puny and insignificant. I said to Frank, "We have to think, however this expedition turns out, what a rare privilege it is to be here now and see this."

He squeezed the top of my shoulder in response and I knew he understood.

"Ken, I don't know why I got so tired on that hike to the flats yesterday. I barely made it to the crevasse and my pulse was over ninety when I got back."

I knew I was the doctor but if Hugh was looking for sympathy, he should have tried someone else. I didn't get past the rise yesterday and my pulse hasn't been below one hundred since I got here.

We were all sitting around in the kitchen tent, but I felt free to consider my own medical situation since the only complaints I heard from others were exhaustion and I didn't believe those anymore. This morning I had awakened with a headache, stuffed nose, and frozen lips, coughing up wet green mucus globs. My pulse was over one hundred. My overnight pee bottle was only half-filled and the color was dark yellow. I got out of breath just dumping it out. After

John and Frank left the tent I took out my stethoscope to listen to my lungs. There were no bubbling noises but one spot had no noise at all—a consolidation that occurs when gunk clogs the air passages and no air can move through. It's a sign of bronchitis when it's due to an irritation like cold air, or of pneumonia if there is evidence of an infection, like for example coughing up green mucus.

On the other hand, the rapid pulse and small quantity of urine could both be due to simple dehydration, the fatigue due to heavy exertion, and the cough due to the dry air. The consolidation was subtle. Maybe it wasn't there at all. When a collection of observations leads inexorably to a conclusion you're not prepared to accept, there is often an inclination to reinterpret the observations. Dealing with the problem would come later.

Actually at that moment I was feeling a little better than yesterday. I hadn't coughed at all since I got up. Though I still wasn't eating, I was cleverly moving the food from one side of the plate to the other so no one would notice and at the same time trying to look alive so I wouldn't be the topic of conversation. I thought I was doing a pretty good job but I didn't impress Todd or Vern. As soon as the others left, they sat down next to me. I knew the jig was up.

"I hope you feel better than you look," Todd said, as an opening.

"Listen," I said, "I might be getting stronger. Let me saddle up today and see what I can do."

On the ice again, with my crampons and pack finally in place I leaned forward on my ski poles and rested standing up. Once I caught my breath, I started off at a pace slow enough to keep my breathing under control. Every few steps my breathing would get ahead of me and I'd have to slow the pace even further. I couldn't get out of first gear and I was getting exhausted. Little snow mounds that I should have stepped over were becoming insurmountable slopes. You would think I was approaching the summit of Mount Everest in a windstorm, and I wasn't even out of sight of the camps yet. A Sherpa from the New Zealand camp next to ours saw me struggling and came out with a bottle. I recognized him as the Sherpa who had passed me in the Cwm a few days ago and who by now I had really begun to believe was a mirage. "Dr. Sab, I bring you hot tea," he said with genuine concern. This was getting embarrassing.

And pointless. It was obvious I was sick and should go down. If I persisted, I'd push myself to total exhaustion and be too weak to make the descent safely tomorrow—a miscalculation that kills a lot of climbers on Everest.

When I turned around, the tents were sickeningly close. I hesitated to take the first step back toward Camp II since it would also be my first step off the mountain. Hopefully I'd recover at base camp but I couldn't be sure I'd ever be back to this mystical place.

This time it was I who sought out Todd and Vern.

"How'd it go?" Vern asked, to be polite as I was sure that with a quick look, the answer was obvious.

"My performance would have to improve for it to be putrid."

"Considering what you looked like when you left the tent this morning." Todd said, "we're surprised you're still alive."

They asked a lot of pointed medical questions and I was surprised at the depth of their knowledge. Uneasily, it occurred to me that though I was the doctor they had far more experience with high-altitude illness than I did. Finally Vern concluded by asking Todd, "What do you think we should do with this patient?"

The question was left hanging since, after all, I was still the doctor. They felt awkward about making the decision so I made it easy. "If I was treating me, I'd send me down."

They both leaned back and relaxed. "A few days of R&R at base camp and you'll be back up here," Todd reassured me.

"Maybe not," said Vern. "I hear there's pretty girls, hot showers, and lots of air down there."

CHAPTER

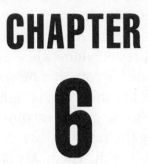

Base camp was a long way down but the morning was sunny, the air was cool and I was feeling better than I had for days. After the initial disappointment, I had a sense of relief that, for the time being at least, my self-imposed pressure was off. Always feeling that I'm not living up to my potential leads to the conclusion that if I don't succeed it's my own fault. But this time it was something beyond my control—I was "sick"—a convenient and comfortable reason to not succeed. I was released from my burden and felt an extra surge of energy.

Skip was designated to accompany me down and we started off at a rapid pace. I was breezing along until we hit the first uphill stretch. Skip didn't even notice it but it made me so tired I had to tell him to stop for a minute so I could catch my breath. After that it just got worse. I was going slower and slower and this was the easy part.

Ahead loomed the rows of wide crevasses that led down to the icefall. I recognized the first one, which was where I got stuck around the bollard on the way up. The fixed rope was still in place and the descent was technically easy, but I

made it look hard. More crevasses followed, and each crossing took longer than the one before. Skip was following
close behind and usually arrived on my side before I finished catching my breath. After one particularly difficult
(for me) crevasse, I rested alone while Skip lingered on the
other side. He shouted across that he was stopping for our
scheduled radio call but the choreography made it apparent
that he wanted me to be out of earshot when he talked to
Todd. Extrapolating the rest was easy. It was already eleven
A.M. and we were still in the Cwm. My slow progress meant
we'd be in the icefall in the afternoon—the riskiest time for
collapses—and we'd be in it a long time. Skip and Todd
would agree on an alternate plan.

Skip came across the crevasse. Before he could say anything I said, "Ken has to stay at Camp One today."

"Yeah," Skip said. "I heard there's a double room available."

The accommodations were as we had left them. A collapsed two-man tent easy to re-erect once we brushed the
snow off, a cache of food and fuel, a cook stove, and an oxygen tank with regulator. I had helped prepare the camp for
an emergency, never for a moment considering that the
emergency could be me.

Out of breath trying to open a can of fruit cocktail, I had
to stop halfway through to rest. Skip got the stove going and
between us we put together a meal. Relaxing in our tent, we
sipped tea and looked out over the silent, vast, empty Cwm.
Accommodations were spartan but the view was spectacular.

No alarm clock was needed here. Our departure time
from Camp I the next day was determined by watching the
slowly brightening sky. Shortly after first light we started off,
timing our descent so there would be adequate illumination
when we hit the icefall. A dull glow was all we needed to finish the Cwm but descending the icefall was technically more

difficult and brighter light was essential. Starting too soon would leave us hanging out at the top of the icefall in the predawn cold waiting for more light. Too late a start and the sun would be melting the most dangerous parts before we got past them.

There was no sign that said "Leaving the Western Cwm," but no sign was necessary. At my feet were an anchor and screw holding a fixed rope that ran several yards along the ice and then disappeared over the edge. Clipping into the rope and checking it twice, I turned around and backed off into the void.

There's no point in worrying about things you can't control once you've made your decision, but we all do it anyway. On the mountain a decision is simpler than at home and easier to accept even when your life depends on it. Once you decide you're going to trust your rope, you stop worrying if it will hold. Rappelling down the side of an ice wall then becomes a very enjoyable experience. There's nothing like dangling from a rope with your feet pressed sideways against a cliff, then pushing off into space riding a pendulum.

This was not the same icefall through which I had come up. Natural forces had already shifted crevasses and ice walls, changing the landscape and showing no regard for our insignificant trail. Some ladders were now uneven and wobbled when we crossed them. Another had become a crumpled ball of aluminum wedged into a crevasse which had obviously narrowed since the ladder was laid across it. Still another was laying across flat, solid ice with no trace left of the crevasse it used to span.

"Wait a minute," Skip called out.

I was about to step across a small crevasse I remembered crossing on the way up.

"That's not a step anymore—it's a jump."

A slight widening of the crevasse had made it dangerous, all the more so because the change was subtle. Skip
planted his ice ax and belayed me by attaching a short
length of rope from the ax to my harness. This would act as
a tether to haul me out if I fell in. He braced the rope and I
jumped across easily. A short jump maybe, but a lot safer
than too long a step.

The more careful Skip was with me, the more annoyed I
became. I knew his concern was a reflection of my poor performance, so his ritual insistence on prudent mountaineering technique began to seem like an insult.

"Nice job, Ken," Skip said as we reached base camp. But
it wasn't a nice job. It had taken me over five hours to get
down the icefall. That's not even a good time for going up.

The camp, with only a skeleton crew of Sherpas, was
nearly empty. All the action was up on the mountain. In the
morning, Skip would be heading back up and I'd be the only
climber here. He volunteered to stay with me a few days but I
said, "No, you belong up at Camp II with the others," trying
to sound selfless. It was depressing enough to be deposited at
base camp. I didn't need someone hovering over me.

He left in the morning after telling me how raunchy I
looked and making me promise to shave and wash up. The
cook-boy brought me a basin of hot water and I took out a
pocket mirror. I hadn't seen my face in two weeks—a liber-
ating circumstance that provides a release most people
never experience. What I saw, though, was disappointing. I
hadn't turned into the hard, bold climber I had been imag-
ining. I still had the same face, only more swollen and more
burned, and Skip was right—I looked raunchy.

My only link to the expedition was through the radio,
and I got word that John was coming down because he was
"too tired." I saw a slow-moving dot coming down the icefall and went out to meet it.

I expected it to be John but it was Jim Young—a New Zealand team member, who took off his gloves as he approached. Thinking this was a polite preliminary to a handshake, I extended my hand but instead of taking it, he opened his palm to show me his blackened fingertips.

Standing right there on the ice I did as careful an examination as I would do in my office—this was my office—and determined that the frostbite was superficial. Jim wasn't easy to reassure. He knew I was a hand surgeon, but he was a professional guitarist.

While I waited for the next dot, Jim headed on down to the New Zealand camp to be treated. I told him to tell Jan that if she needed any help, she should let me know.

The next dot off the icefall was John. He was out of breath and very tired but I told him he looked pretty good.

He said, "Yeah, I feel great. The only reason I came down was because I wanted to breathe."

John sat like a lump in the middle of the medical tent while I examined him. No pulmonary edema, just fatigue. As I was taking the stethoscope out of my ears, I heard a voice outside the tent.

"Ken, it's Jan. Are you in there?"

"Come on in if you don't mind seeing John topless."

She sat on a rolled-up sleeping bag and made herself comfortable.

"Did you see Jim?" I asked, expecting that she had come for some advice.

"Yes, I think Jim will do fine," she replied, "but he told me to, as he put it, 'Go look at Ken because he looks like shit.'"

Too rapidly I was alternating between being the doctor and being the patient. It was getting confusing, but I surrendered my stethoscope to Jan. She listened carefully to my lungs, concentrating a long time on the right base—the lowest lung field—where fluid accumulates first.

"You've got rales and a small consolidation. You've at least got pulmonary edema and probably pneumonia."

She held the end of the stethoscope in place, took the earpieces off, and offered them to me, saying, "If you want a second opinion, listen for yourself."

Doctor's orders: I was sending John down and Jan was sending me down. Base camp is rich in air only by Everest standards. It still has only half what there is at sea level. High doses of air were what we needed, and a trip down to Pheriché, two thousand feet lower, would fill the prescription.

Sitting in a teahouse in Pheriché, I still felt chilled and somewhat weak. We'd been completely out of touch with the expedition for three days. My first night in Pheriché I wrote a letter to Josiane even though there wouldn't be enough time for her to answer me. It was a selfish letter. I told her I had pneumonia and I knew that would frighten her. I wasn't in any danger and there was nothing she could do about it but I needed to share my weakness and self-doubt with someone to whom I was not afraid to be vulnerable. I was preparing myself for the possibility of not succeeding on my grand adventure.

The trail out of town went two ways: uphill was back to Everest, downhill led home; turning downhill would be easy. Still, I knew I couldn't just hike out of my responsibility as the doctor and anyway, the memory of hardship on the mountain was already fading. I still wanted to climb Everest and it would be a few days before I'd have to be brave again. At the end of our three-day convalescence, John and I both turned uphill.

By the top of the flood plain it was obvious that John was a lot better rested than I. We split up so that he could move on ahead. Downshifting for the long slow uphill ride to Loboché, I was still in first gear when I passed a little teahouse and, to my surprise, spotted John's pack outside. We were hardly underway and he had stopped already. Maybe he wasn't as fit as I thought.

As I went to investigate, I passed a guy sitting outside on an oxygen tank leaning against the wall with his head down between his legs. He was wearing a wide-brimmed sun hat and looked like he was taking a siesta. Inside it was dark, but I could make out two people stretched out on the floor drinking tea. I looked for John but instead was amazed to find Skip. Next to him was someone who looked like an older, frightening version of Vern. My head tingled with confusion.

Skip was talking to me but I had to concentrate hard to listen. Nearly the whole team had wiped out trying to go from Camp II to Camp III. They turned back—out of breath, exhausted, and coughing uncontrollably. The next day they were worse, especially Perry, who felt like he was drowning. They had to get themselves off the mountain. Margo and Mike were further up the trail but also heading down. Skip and Vern were here. Perry was the "Mexican" on the oxygen tank outside.

The last time I had seen Perry he was pulling strongly away from me, leading the pack toward the base of Lhotse. Now he needed Skip and me just to stand up and an oxygen tank to keep moving. In the sunlight Vern looked even worse than he had inside. The powerful, fluid animal on the mountain was reduced to taking doddering, uncertain steps and was unable to speak. Skip who had "only" a hacking cough, was leading them down. The ensemble looked like a platoon of wounded soldiers coming back from war.

The two doctors, Matt and Bill, would be at the HRA to greet the wounded but this was a pretty sick pair with more to come. There was no question of our continuing up. John and I made a U-turn and headed back to Pheriché.

Three doctors examining three patients leaves room for nine different opinions. Skip, Vern, and Perry sat slumped forward on benches around the potbellied stove as Matt, Bill, and I did our assembly-line examinations. Namka, the HRA caretaker, served tea and got the fire going. Vern pulled out a jar filled with slimy green bits he had coughed up last night. He thought it would aid in his diagnosis but it was so repulsive none of us would even touch the jar.

Amazingly, the three doctors were in complete agreement. Vern had bilateral pneumonia, Perry had pulmonary edema, and Skip had bronchitis. For Vern, we boiled a pot of water, put a towel over his head, and had him lean over the stove to inhale the warm moist air like he was in a humidifying tent. For Perry, we unrolled the Gamoff bag. It's a body-sized tube that inflates with a foot pedal so that air pressure inside can be elevated above the surroundings. With continuous pumping, a differential pressure can be maintained which is the equivalent of lowering the altitude two thousand feet. The bag was placed behind one of the benches, Perry got in and John volunteered to do the pumping. Skip was given a box of tissues.

Margo and Mike stumbled and coughed their way in, pale and exhausted. They both had pneumonia and in addition, Margo had a permanent painful grimace she couldn't remove from her face. Everyone was slumped down, on benches or on the floor. There was no more room. Namka had to step over and around bodies to distribute more tea.

Margo's grimace finally relaxed and, once she found she could move her mouth, she asked where Perry was. Neither she nor Mike had given thought to John's methodical pumping or to the large orange cylinder lying behind their bench. They both jumped when they learned Perry was inside.

How quickly fortunes can be reversed. This morning John and I felt like the expedition was slipping away from us. This evening, looking at the collection on the benches and on the floor, we seemed more likely to succeed than anyone around us. But the ones who do best in this sport are the ones who stay the healthiest, and those were the ones still at base camp, along with all our Sherpas and all our laser GPS equipment. There was probably enough manpower there to get to the summit and make our measurements but that would be the most dangerous part of the expedition—and the doctor was here, running what sounded like a tuberculosis ward.

Todd and I spoke over the radio. The expedition had broken in two and he was anxious to know when it would be whole again, or at least when I could leave the one piece and rejoin the other. I told him that for now, my patients still needed me. I didn't tell him that for now, I also needed them. They provided a setting where I felt secure and confident of my abilities. I was reluctant to leave my shelter.

One day later Vern felt well enough to play his violin, which he had requested be brought down from base camp along with the medications I had asked for, our camp having better supplies than the HRA. Vern played foot-tapping country music and turned the HRA into a party hall, although some of his captive audience didn't yet seem to be in a party mood.

Two days later Vern was well enough to play his harmonica although, as Bill pointed out, he probably had only five functioning air sacs with which to play it. Using an old guitar left behind by a trekker years ago, Bill teamed up with Vern to take requests. Most of the requests were to "shut up" but they actually played pretty well. There was a chorus of constant coughing in the background, and all together it sounded like a band. After one song, which was followed by weak applause, Bill said, "Okay, that's it. We're ready to take this on the road to Loboché."

It was time for me to take the road to Loboché. I was comfortable where I was but if insulating myself from a threatening environment was the objective, I could have done that better staying home. Instead I was being pulled up the mountain by something else, responding to a call not yet clearly heard—some need to test my limits, to take a risk and see where it led, to seize the chance to make life larger.

But maybe not. Maybe everyday pressures at home create the more threatening environment, pushing me here to escape the drumbeat of responsibility. As they like to say in New Hampshire: "Climbing may be hard but it's easier than growing up."

The route from Pheriché to base camp got a lot longer and a lot steeper. It took me two days to get there. I kept expecting to get into a good rhythm but it never happened. Every time I thought it was getting easier, I realized it was only because I was on a flat spot. Finally I caught a glimpse of prayer flags and I knew the camp was close. Just before I came into full view of the camp inhabitants, I sat down to rest but was unable to gather the strength I needed to make a controlled, triumphant entry. Instead, I staggered into camp looking exhausted and feeling ridiculous. John and I had started out together but he arrived yesterday.

Jan called out to me from her tent. I pretended not to hear and walked on past her camp. She would ask me how I was feeling and I'd be too out of breath to answer. I managed to avoid her but there was no place to hide in my own camp. John came out to greet me, followed by Hugh and Frank, all looking annoyingly healthy. Pete brought me some hot soup—it was obvious I needed something. After the third bowl I felt a little better. I was hoping I was just tired, not still suffering from pneumonia but I could read everyone's mind: I looked worse now than when I left.

Todd tried to cheer me up. "Usually when somebody looks like you, he's dead already."

Pete was more tactful. "Perhaps you're just a little dehydrated."

"Yeah, you're right," I said. "One more bowl of soup and I should have enough strength to collapse."

CHAPTER

Overpowering forces of nature were, as always, sweeping the planet. The tilted Earth, in its orbit around the sun, was bringing the northern hemisphere directly under the sun's rays. The air over the vast Asian continent was heating up, rising into the sky and drawing up, from the huge Bay of Bengal, the wet wind known as the monsoon. It would soon be heading west and north, bringing rain to the plains of India before being forced upward by its collision with the Himalayas. Moving ever higher, the air would cool and the rain become snow. When it reached the heights of Everest, the wind would still be powerful enough to oppose the direction of the jet stream.

Minute beings on the slopes of Everest know they have no control over these forces but dare to try to take advantage of them, scurrying up and down the mountain once the air starts warming but before the monsoon arrives—the interval called springtime. The game they play is to be poised just below the summit when the air masses collide, creating a temporary lull in the jet stream before it changes direction. In the quieter wind, climbers who are strong, healthy, and lucky get to touch the top. Climbers who are only strong and healthy either don't get the chance or don't get back. Failure can mean anything from disappointment to death, and the cause can vary in magnitude from an early monsoon to a broken crampon.

Willing players in this sport of high-altitude mountaineering were checking the weather, their equipment, and themselves with equal intensity, preparing to challenge a mountain that would be entirely indifferent to their fate. Attention to detail is critical, and over the next few weeks each of us had to carry out individual as well as team responsibilities if our expedition was to be successful and safe.

Analysis of wind shifts and snowfall was not my direct responsibility, so I was free to be awed by the daily sprinkling of white powder that covered rocks and tents equally as I made my morning medical rounds. Even though the sick half of my team was still in Pheriché, my practice was booming. As most of the expeditions had not brought along doctors, they were all quite willing to avail themselves of our medical care. I usually made rounds with Jan, and together we treated Argentinean diarrhea, German blisters, Russian hemorrhoids, and international coughing.

Groups of healthy climbers were going "up the hill" every day to fix ropes, build camps, lay in supplies, or maintain the icefall. Sick climbers were being sent down to Pheriché or lower to recover, hopefully better than I had. I was still having trouble walking between the camps to make rounds. Jan invited me for lunch one day—an offer I rarely refused since I enjoyed her company and their food was so much better than ours. Jan was bright and cheery as usual but right away I realized the invitation was an ambush.

Anil, the Indian doctor, and Ricardo, the Spanish doctor, were both there wielding stethoscopes. Including Jan, I was given three examinations. The consensus was I still had rales in my right lung, my pneumonia hadn't cleared, and I needed to go to Namché. It might have made sense medically but if I went that far down now, there would be no reason not to keep going. There wouldn't be enough time to recover and get back. Telling me to go to Namché was like telling me to go to New York. I rejected their advice out of hand, then went back to my tent to actually think about it.

With all our camps in place and the winds on high starting to abate, the door to Everest was cracking open. As it never opens more than a crack, now was the time to pick a summit team and move it into position. I went over the roster with Todd and Pete. The two of them were in the best shape, and Hugh was in the best shape of any of the regular humans. Frank looked tired. Skip was moving easily but was still coughing. John had needed oxygen to slow his pulse down. As for Mike, Margo, Vern, and Perry, they were still the lost legion. We had no idea what shape they'd be in when they got back although I was certain about Vern: With his double pneumonia, he wouldn't be climbing again this season, though I had to admit I couldn't explain his ability to play the harmonica.

One name was conspicuously absent from our discussion: mine. Todd and Pete told me Anil and Ricardo had come to see them today. They were concerned about me and wanted me to go down to Namché. But I presented my case for staying. I wouldn't go any higher unless I felt better and would go down if I felt any worse. Meanwhile we were starting our summit attempt—the most critical time for the expedition—and I wanted to be here. I was thinking more about not missing the action but they took it as an act of altruism and said they'd be glad to have me around.

Excitement filled the camp the next day, which was devoted to getting the first team ready for departure the following morning. I genuinely wanted to do everything I could to help them succeed, but my excitement was waning and it was getting harder and harder to maintain an enthusiastic front.

I finished up my work and wandered back to the mess tent. Todd and Pete were there, surrounded by ice screws, chunks of glass, and what looked like a Tinkertoy set. They were going over the assembly of the laser beacon one more time.

"You guys finally learning how to put this thing together?"

"Yeah. If we can't get it right this time, we're going to read the instructions."

The device was broken down into four transportable sections of aluminum tubing that could be screwed together to make a ten-foot rod. The bottom connected to a long ice screw; the top, to a box with three holes in it. The laser prisms, which looked like traffic lights, screwed into sockets in the holes.

The plan was to screw the rod in as deeply as possible at the exact summit and rotate the box so it faced Namché. Brad Washburn, chief cartographer emeritus for *National Geographic* magazine, would be there with his laser telescope to shoot a beam at the summit. By measuring the angle of the beam and timing how long it took to bounce back, he could calculate the exact height of Everest.

At least that's what Brad told me before I left New York. Looking at this gizmo now, I was asking myself why Brad wanted to put a stoplight on the summit.

Ong-Chu had breakfast ready for us at dawn. We were the second sitting. At 4:00 A.M. he had prepared food for the laser delivery team and had sent them on their way. The camp was empty and quiet after the bustle of the day before.

Lots of expeditions were on the move over the next few days. Skip, as ranking member of our group, handled our radio calls and acted as ambassador to the other camps. Our team was at Camp II, stopped for a rest. The Indians were at Camp III and the Dutch at Camp IV. The Russians were going nowhere.

Skip went to find out why and came back quickly after hearing from them that it was our fault. They had a permit to climb the South Pillar, a very hard route. They couldn't do it so they switched illegally to our route. But they were messing it up—using inferior quality rope and unsafe anchors for the fixed lines, taking our tent sites for themselves, and generally clogging up the way. Todd complained through back channels and got them ordered off the route.

Skip and I were sitting outside with nothing else to do but watch a construction project. Repairs were underway on the mess tent, one side of which had just collapsed after the ice floor underneath it melted away. The Sherpas who were busy reerecting it looked like a circus crew.

It was interesting but not that interesting. After a while Skip said he was going down to the Indian camp for a few minutes. He was gone for hours but I didn't think anything of it until I saw his face when he got back. Something big was going on.

Four Indians had left Camp III to go to Camp IV yesterday. Because they didn't have much oxygen, they had left late—around 11:00 A.M. instead of the usual 8:00 A.M.—in order to spend less time at Camp IV, where you need to breathe oxygen all night. They also weren't adequately dressed (the expedition's clothes just weren't that good) and didn't have any radios. The weather turned bad—cold and very windy. Two climbers made it to Camp IV. One turned back to Camp III. The other was apparently stuck along the fixed ropes somewhere between.

The information came from the Indian who had made it back to III and had borrowed a radio. The only other information the Indian camp had was from a Sherpa who had descended from Camp IV to Camp II today. He said he had seen someone on the ropes at the Yellow Band who wasn't moving. Being a Buddhist, he didn't want to touch a dead body so he moved right past him.

A scheduled radio call with Todd at Camp III was coming up and we all waited to hear if he had any further news. Todd said our entire team had made it okay to Camp III but he had no idea what was going on above. Skip filled him in and Todd said he would go check the Indian tent at Camp III to see if anyone was there.

A few minutes later Todd came back on the radio. Sure enough, he had found one Indian there. Todd brought him back and as we spoke, our team was busy warming and feeding their unexpected houseguest.

The Indian said he had been moving up the ropes behind the expedition leader, Dr. Kalkarni. The two others were ahead of them. There was a high wind, it was very cold and they became exhausted. Kalkarni stopped on the ropes to rest and the Indian, being below him, stopped also. He had the presence of mind, though, to take out his sleeping bag and put it upside down over his head, but only over half his body, since he couldn't unclip from the rope to pull the bag all the way down. Both of them were too exhausted to move and spent the night hanging on the ropes. At about 3:00 A.M. the Indian got some strength back. In the total darkness he was unable to see his teammate but managed to descend to Camp III. With the morning light he looked up the ropes and saw Kalkarni about one hundred meters short of Camp IV. "His arms were moving, not like from the wind." He believed he was still alive.

The story spread quickly through base camp and Rob came to our tent to discuss rescue possibilities. The logical choice was the Dutch, who had two climbers at Camp IV.

"No," Rob said. "I radioed them at Camp Four just now. I told them there were signs of life on the rope. They said they weren't interested."

The next radio message ended the need to mount a rescue. One of the two Indian climbers who had reached Camp IV yesterday descended directly to Camp II today. He told us his partner had staggered into Camp IV exhausted and died of hypothermia during the night. Coming down the ropes in the morning, the Indian passed Kalkarni. He was dead too.

Dinner was pretty grim. Rob stayed to eat with us and share his opinion, which we all wanted to hear, since he was the most respected man in town. He said the accident was avoidable. The Indians left too late, were not adequately dressed, and had used bad judgment. "They should have turned around sooner when the weather deteriorated," Rob concluded, and we all agreed. But four years later we'd be saying the same thing once again, only this time Rob wouldn't be with us—it would be him we'd be saying it about.

When the morning sun hit the icefall I could see a few dots moving down slowly. I had heard that Anil and a few others had gone up early to help their injured teammates and I was sure this must be them coming back. In a few hours they'd be down. Ong-Chu interrupted my observations by asking what I wanted for breakfast. I don't know why. The only choice he had to offer was boiled potatoes on a roll. Supplies were running low.

Later, in my tent, I was doing my best to digest breakfast when I heard the familiar voice of Anil just outside. The cortege was passing through our camp and he broke away to come talk.

"You know we lost two," he said once he entered. "We're bringing the other two down now. One is disoriented, one has got frostbite. The two bodies are still up there; one's still at Camp Four, and the other is on the ropes at the Yellow Band. We wanted to bring them down to Camp Two for cremation but the Sherpas won't touch the bodies. We're going to put them in sleeping bags and drop them in a crevasse.

"You know," he went on after a pause, "Kalkarni and I went to medical school together. He took a personal loan to finance this expedition. Climbing Everest was his dream."

I suppose at this point I should have said something consoling like, "He died doing what he loved." But I couldn't bring myself to say it. Nobody loves hanging from a rope and freezing to death.

To fill the silence I said, "You seem very composed about all this."

He said, "In India, we are used to death."

Our summit team was on the move to Camp IV but we wouldn't have any news for hours. Our base camp team was pretty healthy today, so there was no need for intracamp rounds. Intercamp rounds were another matter.

Jan had asked me to come by to see one of their climbers who had turned around midway through the icefall complaining of rib pain. I timed my visit to arrive just before lunch.

Our patient had a precise area of tenderness between his ribs that I thought was probably an intercostal muscle tear. The New Zealanders were scheduled to go up tomorrow so there was no time to let it heal on its own. He agreed to an injection to try to seal the tear but doubted it would work. He said he would take a walk in the icefall after lunch to see how it felt but we already knew what the answer would be. Jan and I both felt this climber had found the excuse he wanted to not go back up the mountain.

Lunch was tuna and crackers, sliced cheese, french fries, and butterscotch toffee. The Kiwis all looked healthy—what a contrast with our group. Our usual meal was dahlbat, a traditional Sherpa dish made of lentils and rice (sometimes with grass and gravel mixed in) that most of my team members and especially me, found indigestible. Rob thought our poorer condition was due to spending too much time at Camp II and that we would have acclimatized better with more, but shorter, trips. I agreed that might have been better, but each trip through the icefall is a round of Russian roulette.

"Anyway," I concluded, "that's only part of the answer. I think our group is starting to suffer from malnutrition. Pass the tuna please."

In the morning I was glad to step in fresh yak dung. It could only mean one thing: Yaks were around so our supplies had arrived.

"Guess what?" Liz greeted me as I came to the mess tent. "We can start having dahlbat again."

"Yeah, I know," I said, cleaning my boot. "I just stepped in some on my way here."

The trouble with Liz was she actually liked dahlbat and didn't see any reason why we couldn't have it every day like the Sherpas do. I was hoping we'd be seeing some better food now that the yak train had arrived. At least we got toilet paper. The situation had reached the crisis stage and, recently, I had been weighing the ethics of taking some cast padding from the medical supplies.

Not just the yaks arrived today. Also arriving were Vern, looking better, and Margo and Perry, looking about the same. They were just in time to hear the eagerly awaited radio call from our summit team. Todd, Pete, Hugh, and the laser beacon had reached the South Col, (Camp IV,) intact, but coming up on the fixed ropes they had had to pass the body of the Indian still tied in at the Yellow Band. The Sherpas wouldn't let them touch it but, with some difficulty, they were able to clip out and clip in around it. Even so, the Sherpas warned, passing that close could bring bad luck.

After a few hours' rest, the team started out for the summit but the winds above IV were too strong and they had to back all the way down to Camp II to try to wait them out. A little bad luck, but who knows what would have happened if any of our climbers had actually touched the body at the Yellow Band.

The camp seemed crowded over the next few days. We weren't used to all being in the same place at the same time anymore. The summit team had come back, having decided that the high winds weren't going to quit any time soon. They elected to leave the laser beacon at the South Col. Carrying it down and up again would be extra weight. Hopefully someone would be up there again and have the chance to carry it to the summit, or at least to retrieve it. Even though it was only the weather that stopped them this time, Hugh said, "I'm sorry we let you down."

Hugh related how tired he was descending from Camp IV: "As I was coming down I saw somebody else resting against the ropes. I thought that would be a good place to rest too, so I stopped for a minute. Pete came up behind me and said, 'Uh, Hugh, you don't want to rest here.' I suddenly realized I was resting next to the dead body of the Indian. It really shook me up. I tell you, I'm still shook up."

Todd and I collaborated to make up new summit teams. I talked to and examined each climber. Everybody had clear lungs and I thought they all deserved a chance. Perry would have to be watched closely. Once pulmonary edema pops the lungs open, it seems they often don't snap fully shut again. As for Vern, he had recovered from his double pneumonia despite my certainty that he would not. I should have listened more carefully to his harmonica playing.

Todd called a meeting to announce the new schedule. There would be three teams, sent up at one- or two-day intervals. Todd's team would go last. The upper camps were well-stocked and we'd be able to start using oxygen at Camp III. Frank interrupted: "Can I have mine now?"

Todd continued. Once the weather settled, and for as long as supplies lasted, we would keep rotating up the mountain until somebody, or everybody, summited and the laser beacon was installed. Everybody had heard his name called and since we each had a role to play and a chance to summit, the mood in the tent was decidedly upbeat.

Amidst the merriment, Perry realized one name hadn't been called. "What about our doctor?"

Todd answered "Ken is the wild card in all this. He can fit himself in anywhere."

Anywhere or nowhere. I felt essential as the doctor but superfluous as a climber.

The session concluded with Todd announcing that if we got somebody on the summit with the laser, he was going to throw the biggest party we ever saw.

John said "Okay, we all heard that and we're going to hold you to it."

"Yeah," Todd said, "but I didn't tell you where. It's going to be in a teahouse in Loboché."

For now the wind was not cooperating, but the optimistic mood in base camp made the wait tolerable, even pleasant. I liked being in a place where the weather, not the day of the week determined what you did when you got up in the morning. The bad weather enclosed our little circle, forcing us to draw more on the people within. With time on our hands and no easy distractions, long conversations developed between people who would never cross paths outside the mountains.

Like Mike and me. Mike came to my tent to show me a story he had just written about himself as a child and his impressions on moving from Florida to Alaska. He grew up to be a bartender after deciding that selling insurance wasn't for him. His bar became Chilcoot Charlie's, the biggest entertainment complex in Anchorage. When he climbs, he finds sponsors willing to pay one penny for each foot of altitude he attains, then he donates some of the money to the local Police and Fireman's Fund.

"When you own a bar it's a smart idea to have them on your good side. I used to get inspections on Saturday nights to see if my bar was exceeding maximum capacity. Now they come on Tuesday afternoons."

Most of the money Mike collects goes to a mental health charity. One of his children is schizophrenic. He said it was the hardest thing he ever had to deal with. "It's true you can inherit insanity. You get it from your children," he said only half in jest.

Later, Mike unexpectedly came back to my tent and the conversation between the bartender and the doctor continued. He brought his Chilcoot Charlie's banner, an American flag (much smaller than the banner), and trinkets from the police and fire departments. These were the items he was planning to take to the summit and he was eager for me to see them. I had been a good listener.

There was also time to listen to the violin—something I would never do at home. Vern was alone in his tent entertaining himself and I was alone in mine, looking out the door toward Camp I. The music seemed to perfectly match the scene as a fog collected over the icefall.

The mail situation was becoming desperate. Hardly any mail had made it to base camp and we suspected it was all collecting in Namché. Soon we'd be heading up the mountain and it would be good to have a psychological boost before we left. Dorgi was recruited to make a lightning run to the post office in Namché. The deal was, if he could get there and back in three days he could have Todd's sunglasses. Sherpas love sunglasses and he was out of camp before the next dawn.

The other expeditions were stuck like we were and with no telephones, impromptu intercamp visits were the rule. If you wanted to talk to somebody, you had to go see them and spend a little time with them. This was an anachronism that imposed a slower-paced existence, reverting us to an old-fashioned lifestyle with a strong sense of neighborhood.

Jan came to invite me to tea at her camp so I could meet a Sherpa who just arrived today. I shook his hand.

"He wants to say hello to you. Do you recognize him?" she asked. I didn't, so she continued. "He fell in a crevasse at the beginning of the expedition and fractured his skull. This is Pasang-Nuru, the Sherpa you saved."

We shook hands again, this time with a lot more feeling. The semiconscious bleeding patient with the swollen black-and-blue face had been treated in Kathmandu and had come back to rejoin his expedition, looking fresh and fit. Sherpas don't easily use words to say thank you, but all the thanks I needed was expressed in his smile and in the tight grip with which he held my hands.

It was an easy decision to stay for lunch, but I wasn't the only visitor. As we were talking, four people came in surrounded by a lot of commotion. It was the French expedition. I had heard a lot about them but this was the first time I saw them: three guys and one very attractive girl. They were "going light." In theory that means moving very rapidly by taking few supplies. In practice, though, it often means "borrowing" supplies from other expeditions. In fact, they had come because the girl had broken her crampon and they had no spare.

Rob went off to try to find a pair that would fit her and she sat down next to me, happy for a chance to speak French to someone new. Her name was Chantal Mauduit and though she was a natural coquette, she was also a serious climber. The group was heading down to Pheriché for a few days of R&R before coming back up for a summit attempt. Rob found the crampons too quickly and the entire group sprang up and left the tent, taking all the commotion with them.

Later, I told Todd I had met the nice-looking French girl.

"Yeah," he said. "Chantal is very French. Watch out for me; I'll give her as much oxygen as she wants."

Yesterday we had heard that "the weather was good upstairs," so early this morning Skip, Vern, and Mike started off toward the summit. There was hopeful anticipation in the camp. Pete, Perry, Frank, and Margo were planning to leave tomorrow. The more I thought about it, the more I thought I could try to go up with them. They were the weakest team so I'd have the best chance of keeping up. Especially with Margo—she still looked terrible.

A few hours later Margo came running to my tent.

"Something's wrong with Mike at Camp Two."

I quickly put my clothes on and ran with her to the mess tent thinking I'd have to give some kind of emergency instructions to save Mike. Todd was on the radio speaking to him very routinely and was surprised to see me. Mike's cough had gotten worse and he wanted me to send up some cough syrup but it was nothing that couldn't wait until later. Margo had overreacted. She was very nervous about going up tomorrow.

She admitted as much when I took her aside to talk. Like Mike, her cough also had gotten worse. She was upset and wanted me to check her out. In the medical tent I listened to her lungs. There were diminished breath sounds and crackling noises on the right. As gently as I could, I said, "They don't sound as good as they did a few days ago."

She understood what I was telling her. She would be scratched from the team tomorrow and knew there wouldn't be another chance. She started to cry and leaned against me. I put my arm around her and she cried some more. She had had a rough time growing up as a rich girl in Greenwich, Connecticut, surrounded by boys, booze, and drugs. One day she woke up on the floor of someone's house and resolved to use mountains to climb out of her miserable life.

Climbing had given her the vehicle to rise above her addictions and in the process she had reached the top of the highest mountain on each continent except Asia. Summiting Everest would have made her the first American woman to complete all seven peaks. She could deal with her own disappointment, but being somewhat of a celebrity in rehab circles, she would have a harder time dealing with the disappointment of people who looked to her for inspiration.

I was eliminating any chance Margo had to climb Everest. It was a huge responsibility. I wanted to make sure I was right and I also wanted some backup in case Margo would later come to doubt my decision.

"Look, Margo, let's go see what Jan thinks."

Margo liked the suggestion. At least it would change the scene, and maybe she'd prefer another woman to talk to.

All I said to Jan was, "Examine Margo and tell me what you think."

She listened to her lungs carefully, then said, "You can't go up tomorrow."

Margo's last hope was gone and though I could feel her disappointment, I also felt relief. My opinion had been confirmed and it made the decision easier. Margo cried on Jan's shoulder and said, "I'm coming back next year even if I have to mortgage my house to do it."

During dinner, our mailman, Dorgi, returned from Namché. He was very proud to have made the roundtrip in three days. Even today's all-day snow hadn't stopped him from keeping his appointed rounds. We heartily congratulated him for getting back in time to give us our mail before we left for the summit.

"Where did you put it, Dorgi?"

"No mail."

"What do you mean 'no mail'?"

"I come to Namché late. Post office closed. If I stay Namché for post office next day, I no be back in three days so I come back right away."

It all made perfect sense to him and he was confused by our befuddled reactions. He sincerely felt he had done what we had asked of him. Todd gave him the sunglasses.

I decided to leave the next morning with Pete, Perry, and Frank. Before going to sleep that night I performed my secret ritual. I took out my collection of notes (the first one from the airplane plus all the "hidden ones" that I'd discovered so far), looked at the family picture, smelled a perfumed handkerchief into which I tucked the little stuffed dolls, then put it all in the top pocket of my windbreaker. I'm traveling light but those are essentials.

CHAPTER

My tent was dark, cold, and silent, but I came instantly awake at 4:00 A.M., responding to some internal timer that went off precisely at the prearranged wake-up time. Outside, there were lights of various colors: An opaque blue light shone through the fabric of the cook tent as Ong-Chu prepared breakfast. A few yellow lights moved in seemingly random horizontal patterns as climbers with headlamps got themselves ready. An orange flame was making juniper smoke. Overhead were millions of white points. The lights, though still overwhelmed by the darkness, were enough to set the scene: Skies were clear above an awakening base camp.

Like so many times before, we were heading into the icefall but this time we were aiming for the summit. After two months on the mountain it all came down to the next few days. I had no special feeling other than to wonder whether or not I will have climbed Everest the next time I saw base camp.

The icefall was the same, meaning nothing was the same. Though we saw no movement, evidence of movement was everywhere. Deep cracking noises accompanied scenes of crumpled ladders. We were in the bowels of the mountain.

The serac with the embedded orange tent that had marked the top of the icefall had collapsed, and the tent was now lying tattered and splattered across the route like a finish-line flag for Camp I.

If the day had ended here, I would have been okay but this was only the halfway point. We were continuing on to Camp II after a short break. I was tired and cold and needed to blow my nose. The delicate smell of the handkerchief I took from my pocket temporarily overpowered my harsh surroundings and, for a moment, transported me home.

A perfumed handkerchief, however, doesn't make up for a lack of acclimatization. The others had been up here twice—me, only once. The Cwm was about one-third too long for me. Just below the final slope I stopped to finish my water, and Pete, coming up from behind as the sweeper, stopped with me. It would have been easy to gaze up the Lhotse face to Camp III at that moment, but I was careful not to. That part of the route seemed so impossibly long last time when I was here with pneumonia. This time I was exhausted and didn't want to see it the same way again. I'd look at it tomorrow after I was rested and maybe it wouldn't give such a fearful impression.

Frank and Perry greeted me at Camp II with handshakes and hugs, saying, "We all made it." Perry took off my crampons while Frank brought me some tea. I had just about gathered enough strength to get up from my rock and go to my tent to collapse when Pete said, "Ken, a few of the Sherpas want you to look at them."

I couldn't believe it. I was wiped out. I told Pete, "No tent calls. Have the Sherpas come to my rock."

They came. I treated one cough, one sore throat, and one back pain and then crawled to my tent.

While it was true we all made it, this was the weakest group and I was the slowest of the slow. Frank and Perry thought it was a great achievement for me to get to Camp II at all. It might be relatively good for someone getting over pneumonia, but Mount Everest deals in absolutes.

Everyone except us was on the move the next morning. We had a rest day, but Todd and Hugh were coming up from base while Skip, Vern, and John were going from III to IV. Mike was also at III but he was heading down.

He came into Camp II weak and tired, coughing continuously. He had taken some of the codeine syrup I sent up for him two days ago and carried the rest to Camp III, into ever colder and drier air. The cough worsened and the syrup froze. He thawed the bottle as best he could and drank it. It was an icy slush that irritated his throat, provoking even more coughing. My medicine had made him worse.

Mike didn't need me to tell him his expedition was over. This was his second try on Everest and he had promised his wife it would be his last. He said, "When you set your sights so high, you have to be prepared to accept disappointment."

Perry asked, "Why don't you try again next year?"

Mike said, "To do that, I first have to get a new wife."

Perry was my other patient. He was a lot stronger than I was but I was worried about him. He had had pulmonary edema two weeks ago and once you've been hit, you're at greater risk to get it again, no matter how clear your lungs sound.

I put my stethoscope down so we could talk. I encouraged him to tell me about his ten-month-old daughter. He didn't need much prompting and was quick to show me a set of pictures. As we looked at the last one I said, "Let's not forget what's important here. At the first sign of trouble, you are off the mountain."

Although it had been snowing all day, Todd and Hugh got up from base camp in good time. Skip, Vern, and John made it to Camp IV—they'd be going for the summit that night. My team was preparing to try for III tomorrow. Mike was getting ready to go home.

Todd and I were in the mess tent. He was adjusting his crampons and I was meticulously packing a duffel bag with personal supplies for Camp III that a Sherpa would bring up for me tomorrow. Mike came in carrying his banner, his flag, and his trinkets. He asked Todd, "Can you take these to the summit? It would mean a lot to me."

Todd said, "Sure. If I can make it up there, your stuff will too."

Mike smiled but looked dejected. What a difference from the enthusiasm in my tent just a few days ago.

After dinner Pete felt compelled to make a speech. "I've been to the summit twice, but it took me five tries to get there the first time. You've all put a lot of resources and effort into this, but Everest doesn't care. Safety is first. Slow means dangerous. We'll have turnaround times tomorrow. If you haven't reached certain points by certain times, you have to back down. We've seen what happens when people push the limits. We are not going to do that. We want everyone back in one piece. The mountain will always be there."

Pete wanted us to be mentally ready, but I wasn't sure I was. The route to III was in plain sight, but all day I had avoided looking at it. There's a difference between respecting a mountain and being fearful of it. Respect creates a standard that you can reach within yourself to match. Fear opens a tap that will drain your energy as surely as pneumonia. I had been weakened by fear or by pneumonia, but either way I had failed to overcome the weakness and so far was unable to generate the positive attitude I needed to climb Mount Everest.

"John is snow blind!" was my wake-up call. Todd was outside my tent on the radio to Camp IV. They were preparing to leave for the summit but John said his eyes were burning and he could see only blurry images. Yesterday, while going to Camp IV, oxygen leaking from his mask continually fogged his goggles. The sun wasn't too bright so he took the goggles off. He didn't feel anything then but now he said it was the worst pain he'd ever had.

I told Skip to put tetracaine, a numbing solution, in his eyes and then patch them closed. I reassured John that the blindness, although often total, was temporary. It was a sunburn of the corneas—the transparent windows that let in light—and it would heal by itself in a few days. He'd have to stay at Camp IV until the others got back. There was no question of a summit attempt for him now.

Though I had been awakened from a sound sleep, I discovered it was only midnight. I went back for a few more hours of rest, then reawoke for breakfast and prepared to take my first step toward Camp III. Last time I was here I hadn't reached the New Zealand camp after fifty minutes and had to turn around. This time I was there in twenty minutes. As I passed by, I recognized the Sherpa who had been my mirage in the Cwm and my tea server when I had been too weak to continue. This time he held his hand high and said, "Yes, Dr. Sab!" I was off to a good start.

Perry and Frank had left a few minutes ahead of me but I caught up to them as they were crossing a ladder. While I held the safety line taut, I took a hard look at the route to Camp III for the first time since my retreat. It didn't seem so impossibly far, and I was encouraged.

The flats sloped up toward the long snow ramp that rose to the first fixed rope. The ropes were invisible from here, but they led straight up the face of Lhotse to Camp III. I knew where the camp was situated, though at this distance it was invisible too.

As the slope turned gradually upward, breathing became harder and my movements were slower, as if increased gravity was drawing strength out of me. Frank was going even slower and dropped behind me. He looked so tired that when he fell in a hole, I thought for a second he had collapsed, but he still had the strength to smile. I was keeping my face expressionless to save energy.

Pete dropped back to stay with Frank, and soon the two of them were out of sight as Perry and I continued on together. I was going slowly and I didn't want Perry holding back to stay with me. Several times I said, "Why don't you go ahead a little bit." He would spurt ahead a few yards and then rest until I caught up. Although he professed to not have much more power than I, I suspected he didn't want to leave me alone.

Pete reappeared without Frank and fell in behind us as we plodded on without stopping or even turning our heads. From behind we heard Pete say, "He was too tired and turned back," but the explanation was superfluous.

The quiet was broken by an excited radio call. Skip and Vern had just reached the summit. I felt obliged to say "great" and put my hand up in the air, but my show of excitement was really just a show. I wasn't jealous. It was just that we were in our own world here—far away and very detached from what was going on at the summit.

At the snow ramp the route steepened and the air I inhaled seemed to stop halfway down my throat. I had to slow my pace even further to gain time to force the air all the way down after each step. The ramp was enormous but I knew for sure it had an end. I had seen it, so I resolved to keep moving until I reached it. I was already much further than I had gotten last time and I was always able to take at least one more step.

Perry, Pete, and I moved along in silence, each lost in his own thoughts. I don't think a single word was spoken for the entire length of the ramp. Then, out of the quietude, the first fixed rope suddenly appeared—the passage to the upper reaches of Everest. Pete said, "Let's take a break here."

It didn't seem odd to me then, but this was the first time in two days of climbing that Pete had ever suggested stopping. He didn't say anything right away. We all took long drinks from our bottles. I was a little uneasy about our rate of progress and his lack of urgency to get started again, so I said lightly, "How are we doing?"

He took the opening. "You really want to know? I'll be honest. We're moving slower than I'd like. It's taken us three and a half hours to the ropes. The maximum time should be three. Not that the half hour is critical, but you've been slowing down, you look tired and you're out of breath. I realize it's your first time up this high but the others, even on their first run, did it in two and a half to three hours. A time I'd like to see on the summit run is one and a half to two hours. And the hardest part of the climb is just starting. The ropes require a lot more energy. At the rate we're going, we won't get to Three for at least six more hours and that's too late. It's dangerous to be on the ropes that long and that late. You're doing better today than you did coming up to Two and maybe if you had another week to be over the pneumonia, you'd be able to do it, but right now you just don't have the strength. I don't think it's safe for you to continue. This is a very unforgiving mountain. It's very hard for me to tell you this. I hope you understand that as your friend I'm doing what's best for you."

Up to that moment I had felt like it was no big thing if I didn't climb Everest. It wasn't a lifelong dream, just a tough challenge with long odds. I was able to soften the blow for the others who had been eliminated, but the sudden realization that it was over for me hit me hard. I looked at the first fixed rope and thought, I'm not going to see what's at the other end.

I started to cry but the tears were contained by my dark goggles. I didn't say anything; my voice would have cracked if I tried.

There was a long, motionless silence. I knew I had to be the next one to speak, so finally I said to Pete, "I have to respect your judgement—no one knows this mountain better than you. I know I could get to Camp Three (I needed to believe that for myself) but if you think the margin of safety is too thin, it's your call to make."

Pete said, "If you had another week or two to recover, it might be different. You've shown tremendous determination to come this far after the pneumonia. You just needed more time."

There was a pause while I got control of myself again. I said, "I understand. You're doing the right thing."

I couldn't say any more.

We were all standing now. Pete and I hugged each other—a real hard hug—and then I hugged Perry. I put my pack on, turned around, and headed down the mountain—at a pretty good rate. I knew they were watching me and I wanted to go out with style.

Now that I was alone I started to cry again. I hadn't realized how much of my ego was invested in this and didn't understand why that should be. After all, I was the respected doctor and even more, the beloved husband and father—unassailable achievements from which to draw strength—yet I felt my self-esteem to be deeply wounded by this mountain. The consolation prize was the esteem accorded to me as the expedition doctor and perhaps that was a greater prize than the summit, but right then it didn't seem to be enough. My reaction didn't fit my self-image, and I was surprised by my vulnerability.

The crying lasted a few minutes and then I was over the shock. As I moved down the snow ramp, I started to get my equilibrium back. It would have been great to summit Everest, but far more awaited me in the direction I was headed now. By the time I reached the flats, I was settled: It was a huge mountain but insignificant compared to what I had at home.

I didn't expect to be back in camp so soon. I took a seat in the mess tent with Todd and Frank. Todd was proud some of our team had summited. He knew his chance was coming. Frank was depressed. He knew his chance was gone.

While we were talking I realized, with a start, that I was sitting on the duffel bag of supplies that was supposed to be brought to Camp III for me. It had never left the tent. Though I suspected why it hadn't, I asked Todd for an explanation. He admitted that he thought I wouldn't make it and he didn't want to waste a Sherpa trip. That made me feel worse than I already did. He said if he had heard I was doing well, he would have sent the bag up a little later. I guessed it made sense from an expedition point of view but I felt betrayed.

This was the most dangerous time for the expedition, so I decided to stay put at Camp II the next few days. It would be more exciting to be here than to be socializing at base camp. More important, it was where I would be the most valuable, and right now I needed to feel valuable. My decision was hailed as another great selfless move by the doctor.

I went back to my tent to get installed. I didn't have the heart to unpack the duffel bag that I had organized and arranged with so much care yesterday. Instead I took out the stuffed dolls and family pictures from my pocket. They all looked the same as when I zipped them in this morning. Nothing had changed.

One by one the summiters came back into camp. I patted each of them on the back and did the congratulations thing. When it was Frank's turn, he did even less. It wouldn't be fair not to give them their moment. I did my best to be the audience they deserved, though my enthusiasm was hollow.

My reaction for Vern was more genuine. I was awed by his comeback. His pneumonia had been much worse than mine and I hadn't been able to do it.

John and Skip came in together. John was still barely able to see, so Skip had to lead him down the fixed ropes all the way. John was exhausted, physically and emotionally. He was on the verge of crying as he said, "It was close and if the Big Guy wanted me to make it, I would have made it."

The others went down to base camp the next morning, some bringing "summit rocks" for their children. I could only collect "interesting stones from Camp II" for mine, as I waited three more days to see the final summit team safely back. I felt stupid to still be here, but then I reminded myself I was the doctor.

Because the Cwm has a dogleg and radio signals can't bend, Camp II can talk to Camp IV or to base camp but base camp and Camp IV can't talk to each other. I was the only link among the three groups. In the morning I made a call to Camp IV to see if the summit team was underway and Perry answered. The others had left but he "wasn't feeling right" and told them at the last minute to go without him. He was just waiting there until they got back.

I asked him what "not feeling right" meant. He said when he lies down he has trouble breathing. He said it calmly but at my end of the radio it went off like an alarm.

His pulmonary edema was coming back. I never should have let him go, flashed through my mind. Over the next twelve hours it could progress to unconsciousness and even death. The summit team could easily take another twelve hours to get back, and by that time Perry's condition could deteriorate so drastically that getting him down would be difficult or impossible—or even unnecessary.

Telling Perry to stand by, I pointed the radio down to base camp and spoke to Vern. He understood the situation immediately. Pemba, one of our strongest Sherpas, was the only other person left at Camp IV and he would have to come down tied to Perry in case he deteriorated on the ropes. Vern also suggested the possibilities of giving Perry nifedipine, dexamethasone, and oxygen. He was careful to say it very respectfully, making it clear that I was in charge. I appreciated his approach and was impressed with his level of knowledge about the drugs. I told him I already had Perry taking the nifedipine, as well as an extra dose of diamox, and he would be coming down on oxygen. Perry's speech was clear and he was able to handle the radio so his coordination was good and the dexamethasone wasn't needed—at least not yet.

Vern and I had managed to have a thoughtful, intelligent conversation over a walkie-talkie, not an easy thing to do, especially since I interrupted him several times, reversing antenna direction to make sure Perry was preparing to leave. Perry had endless questions, some of which I had to relay to Vern and then relay back the answers. The questions got less and less important. Finally he asked me to ask Vern if he should melt ice before he left so the summit team would have some water when they got back. At that I said, "Perry, would you please just get the hell out of there. Now!"

He said, "Okay, okay" and got off the radio.

Perry could probably get down in about six hours—maybe less if his condition improved with the lowering altitude. If he got worse though, he'd be completely exhausted by the end and Pemba might need help getting him across the flats. Reluctantly, I reached the conclusion that it would be a good idea for me to go partway up to meet them.

It would be a slow trip. I hadn't eaten much lately. Not having any appetite nor much food around, and thinking my only climbing would be down, I had developed the obstinate attitude that I didn't have to eat anymore, so I wouldn't. This makes sense only to five-year-olds and people who stay too long at Camp II.

I waited two hours to leave, slowly packing a kit of emergency supplies including injectable drugs, chocolate bars, and hot tea. I tried to time my departure so I'd meet them at the bottom of the snow ramp. Leaving too soon would be dangerous. It was very cold out. I didn't want to stand around and wait.

I needn't have worried about that. I was slower than I expected. I couldn't get enough air as I walked and had to stop every few steps to resupply. The sky was overcast and it started to snow. I thought I was nearing the top of the flats but I wasn't sure. Visibility was becoming really poor and I was afraid I was getting lost.

Out of the opaque curtain ahead of me two gray silhouettes appeared. One was treading lightly, the other plodding along with an uneven step. I was really glad to see them, not sure at this point who was rescuing whom.

Perry was overwhelmed to see me and fell into my arms. I sat him down in the snow and took off his oxygen mask so he could drink the tea I poured him. Pemba sat also and drank a polite amount, but Perry drank nearly all of it. He was dehydrated and weak but breathing okay and still warm and coordinated. Tea and chocolate would do it for now; no need for the meds. Perry got up and Pemba led us both back to camp.

Safe and sound. Perry was going to be okay. He was resting next door in his tent and I was resting in mine—lying on top of my sleeping bag, exhausted but exhilarated. The fatigue would pass but the chance I was given to help Perry would leave me with one timeless cosmic moment: Perry told me that when he was coming over the slope and saw somebody waiting below, he said to himself, "Please God, let that be Ken."

And it was.

The last summit team was the most successful. They were the strongest and most deserving. Todd had been trying to climb Everest for ten years and this was his third try. For Pete this was his third success—the only non-Sherpa to summit that many times. And he had completed the installation of the laser reflector, screwing in the three prisms and sinking the whole unit in deeper, though never hitting bedrock. The ice cover on the summit was thicker than we thought or else very possibly it was skewed by the wind so that the ice summit was not overlying the rock summit. An intriguing idea to consider later, but right now the reflector was on the summit, aimed toward Namché and waiting for Brad.

My life is on the other side of the icefall, and it was time to go home. It occurred to me that this descent might be the last time I ever passed this way and I felt obligated to stop and appreciate the otherworldly beauty I had been allowed to see. But ethereal thoughts were quickly crowded out by the imperatives of getting through the icefall.

The question I had asked myself the last time I started up was whether or not when I returned to base camp I would have summited Everest. The answer was no. The mess tent was festooned with pink toilet paper, and a big sign that said *Congratulations* listed the names of the summiters. A smaller sign had my name on it, and next to it was written *Expedition Doctor and Saint.*

Spirits were high. Todd recalled how he resisted temptation on summit day. He had thought about installing the laser reflector just below the South Summit instead of at the real summit. The measurements would then have shown Everest to be about one thousand feet lower and K2 would be proclaimed the highest mountain in the world. Todd said he didn't think Brad, *National Geographic,* or the Nepalese would find it very funny, but it would have been the greatest hoax in exploration history.

Ong-Chu baked a cake for the occasion and brought it out proudly. He had used a mix, then added his own touch by decorating the top with sliced tomatoes. The scene was all handshakes and hugs, congratulations to the summiters and heartfelt comments to me about what a great job I had done. I accepted the accolades as graciously as I could. Yeah, great doctor I thought, but I couldn't even get to Camp III.

CHAPTER

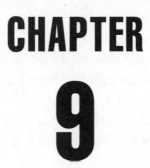

When I came back to New York it was springtime; the greens and the flowers were more vibrant than ever. I saw my life more vividly, too—renewing my feelings for Josiane as they were when we first got to know each other. I was content with all the familiar things around me and I delighted in simple pleasures like going to the bathroom without having to put my boots on.

I said that no matter how high I got on the mountain, the experience would be worth it, and it was. I had entered that far-off world of adventure and excitement and, surprisingly, had found people there just like me. It was a geographic and social assortment that I would otherwise never have gotten to know in the larger society where I have more choices and less time. The prolonged confinement compelled us to get to know each other and, like a child with only a few toys to play with, I formed a greater attachment to each one. I found a lot more than appeared on the surface. Bonds of friendship formed swiftly, strengthened by the hardships we endured and the emotions we shared.

Everest was more than the mountain; it was who I climbed it with.

I had formed friendships built on trust, respect, and even mutual admiration with Todd and Pete, both of whom would take on hero roles in 1996, and with Frank, who would be one of the unwilling players in that disaster. I had renewed my six-year-old friendship with Rob Hall. And I had opened a medical practice with Jan, a skillful doctor who enjoyed practicing on Mount Everest almost as much as she enjoyed being with Rob.

It took two weeks for the currents inside me to calm enough so I could return to work. Fears about losing my practice turned out to be totally unfounded. Business picked up immediately and soon I was busier than ever. My trip had brought great notoriety and my referral base expanded. New patients would tell me their doctor had told them to "Go see my friend, the mountain climber," though in many cases the doctor was someone I had never even met.

As the crowning achievement, I brought back Nima Tashi. Long Island Jewish Medical Center, the hospital where I do most of my surgery, was immediately taken with the idea of helping the needy Sherpa; no arms needed to be twisted. Doctors, nurses, and administrators all volunteered their time and services and were enthusiastic to be part of the effort. Pete collected funds to pay Nima Tashi's airfare, although I suspect Pete, himself, provided most of those funds. After undergoing the world's most sophisticated tests, we determined that the combined effect on an ankle of falling three hundred feet and being walked on while dislocated for over a year was to destroy the joint totally. An ankle has two parts—an upper hinge for front-and-back motion to step up and down, and a lower part for side-to-side motion to accommodate uneven terrain. Both functions were critical for life in the mountains and both were completely gone. Nima Tashi's ankle would have to be fully fused—made into a solid L-shaped piece. His leg would bend only at the knee, forefoot, and toes, but he'd be able to walk, and he'd be without pain.

The surgery was planned and carried out with Dr. Ron Light, a friend and former junior resident of mine who had gone on to become an orthopedic trauma specialist. Our children helped out, too. During Nima Tashi's stay, they decorated the bare walls of his room with pictures of what they imagined life was like in the strange place where he came from—drawings of mountains, stone houses, and yaks.

Pete hung around New York before, during, and after surgery to act as interpreter and caregiver. The whole event caught the imagination of New York television and newspapers, and Nima Tashi was interviewed repeatedly. Being shy and not knowing what to make of all this attention, he wasn't able to say much, but Pete's liberal translations smoothed the way. When asked his impression of life in the United States and the help he was receiving, Nima Tashi would reply, "Ramro," which to me means "good." Pete's translation, however, was, "Nima Tashi wants everyone to know how much he loves America and how deeply he appreciates the care he is receiving here." I never argued with Pete's version. He spoke much better Nepali than I did and he was a better diplomat, too.

During the six months it took for Nima Tashi's ankle to fuse solidly, he was shuttled around the country to stay as a guest in the homes of various American climbers who had been with him in the Himalayas. The Immigration and Naturalization Service asked me to guarantee that Nima

Tashi would be going back to Nepal someday. I assured them he had no intention of staying on as an indigent immigrant when, at home, he not only had a family, he was a celebrity. When he was fully healed, he went back to Nepal, walking through the airport with a surprisingly mild limp and holding the children's pictures from the hospital rolled up under his arm. There was a special place he wanted to put them, he told me, but it would be two years before I found out where. I advised him once more that he'd be able to herd yaks and plant potatoes but he'd never be able to climb again. He patiently and respectfully said yes to everything I told him, but he had no intention of following my advice.

I had gone to the mountain unsure of my ability to handle high-altitude emergencies, but was perceived as being competent right from the start. That perception, I felt, had developed into reality by the time the expedition was over. I had been fully tested as a doctor and I was satisfied, even proud, of my performance, but I hadn't come near being tested as a climber. I didn't want to believe my limit was Camp II.

Josiane was disappointed when I returned, but not in the way I expected. She didn't care that I hadn't summited. She was disappointed that I wanted to go again. Everest had stolen a lot of time from us. Events had come and gone without me. She had worried over and resolved family problems that I didn't even know about—little bits of their lives that I would never share.

It wasn't just the three months I was away; it was the year I had spent planning it—giving my attention to Everest rather than to us. She wished now that I would turn back to her and the family. Uneasily, she was beginning to think there wasn't enough to keep me at home.

I saw it differently. My personal expedition was unfinished. I had set a goal and wanted either to achieve it or find out that I couldn't; either way would be satisfying. I wasn't obsessed with Everest, but it had brought out the best in me and I didn't want it to stop now. I was aware of the impact on my family but dismissed the selfish nature of the undertaking with the argument that my total time with Josiane and the children was still greater than what most husbands and fathers spend with their families. My preparation time came from shortening hours at work, not home. True, Everest preoccupied my thoughts, but I reasoned that was no different than any other professional who takes his work home with him in his mind.

The danger had to be reconsidered as well. Three Indian climbers had died while I was there. They brought realism to the abstract concept of risk, but they weren't part of my expedition and I didn't know them. It had happened to "them," not "us." I had the belief, which Josiane shared as well, that people like Rob, Todd, Pete, and me could control the risk. That belief, however, was based on the assumption that risk was controllable.

Josiane agreed to let me go back a second time, at first reluctantly, but then with some enthusiasm, albeit less than the first time. I didn't get much past Camp II on the second try either, and there followed a third and a fourth try over a total of five years. Instead of a once-in-a-lifetime event, Everest had become a way of life. Josiane never told me not to go, though she found it harder and harder to gather her enthusiasm each time. She felt I was submerging my other interests, and my time at home was being reduced to interludes between expeditions.

There wasn't much discussion of danger anymore. Though the risks of Everest hadn't lessened, our perception of them had. As a doctor, I saw the phenomenon often: An experienced laborer who worked with dangerous equipment gradually relaxed his vigilance until he showed up in the emergency room with a severed hand. Familiarity, and prolonged exposure without incident, leads to a loss of appreciation of risk. And so it was that with each successive safe return from Everest, our sense of danger receded.

CHAPTER
10

The cold woke me up. In the dark I didn't know where I was or what was holding me here. As my head slowly cleared, however, the immediate mystery was solved. I was at base camp zipped into my sleeping bag, but I was certain that if I didn't fully awaken, I would fall asleep again and be back home when I really woke up. Instead I chose to stay where I was. I unzipped my sleeping bag, then unzipped my tent, emerging from both my shelters.

The larger mystery of what was holding me here would be harder to solve. It was 1995—my third trip. In two previous seasons, I had been on Everest a total of five months and now I had returned for at least two more. I knew that much of the time I would be cold, tired, and scared but paradoxically, Everest had come to seem like a protected place. It was a haven where I could lead a simpler life. Though death was always around us, it was in the background, happening to other people, not my friends, not my little group.

This year, as in previous years, I had renewed old friendships and made new ones in this isolated village called Everest Base Camp. Todd, Pete, and Frank were back, as well as our sirdar, Lakpa-Rita, and Ong-Chu, our cook. Newer additions were Wally Berg, an avalanche ski patrolman and mountain guide from Colorado, and Jim Williams, a geologist and mountain guide from Wyoming. Rounding out our group were some amateur climbers like myself including: Todd "Mook" Hoffman, an easy-to-like businessman whose personality undoubtedly contributed a great deal to his success; and Lily Leonard, whose excitement for adventure contrasted nicely with her training as a research biochemist. All together, it was a collection of levelheaded but somewhat aberrant people who were now making their way to the mess tent.

What was bringing us together this morning was a meeting to plan for the installation of some new GPS equipment at various points on the way to the top of the mountain. But, in a larger sense we were together because of a personal challenge each of us felt to try to reach the summit. That motivation, however, would seem a lot less compelling once death penetrated our little circle.

"Very good, Dr. Sab, Camp Three," said Kami as I entered the mess tent. He poured me some tea and gave me the thumbs-up sign. Kami was a new Sherpa in camp. I checked carefully: He wasn't just an old face with a new hat. Kami came from the same village as Lakpa-Rita, who had picked him as his protegé. He was given a job as cook-boy this year but was young and ambitious and wanted to work his way up one day to climbing Sherpa or sirdar. He was learning English, being helpful wherever he could, and seemed to be on the fast track.

The meeting had already started and I regretted being late, not because I missed anything, but because all the spots near the propane heater were already taken. We had been on Everest for five weeks already. The past few days we had spent high up on the mountain completing our second foray to build the upper camps and set up the route to the summit. This was our first day back in base, and maybe my confusion upon awakening this morning was due to oxygen intoxication from too much air. The trip had been successful for the team as well as for me personally. I reached Camp II without pneumonia or even undue shortness of breath. Feeling strong, the distance between II and III seemed long but not impossible any more. Whether my confidence came from better health or my strength was due to a better attitude, there was enough within me to reach Camp III. The Lhotse Face no longer intimidated me.

I was feeling positive and so was Todd. He said the weather continued to look good—cold and light snow don't count. There wasn't much wind or fog, and the jet stream was abating with no sign of the monsoon yet. The plan was to rest down here for about three or four days— eat, drink, relax, get our strength up, and then go for the top. If the weather held and everything went right, we could be on the summit in ten days. The possibility was exciting. In a few days, for the first time, I would be part of a summit team.

Incredibly, Nima Tashi would be part of that team as well. He had scrupulously followed my advice in the United States but then totally ignored it once he returned to Nepal. He went back to climbing his first week home and, despite his rigid ankle, soon regained his skill, strength, and prestige. His gratitude to me was limitless, and though Lakpa-Rita had hired him as a team climber, he was doubling as my personal Sherpa, attentive to little details like adjusting my pack straps and checking my rope. I was the only climber on Everest with valet service.

As the meeting broke up, the sun suddenly came out and I wanted to take advantage of it. My goal for the day suddenly became to take a shower and change my underwear. It had taken a few seasons but finally we had a shower that worked well. It was Liz's legacy. I was about to ask Ong-Chu for shower water when he came to me suggesting a starting time. Either he read my mind or I smelled worse than I thought.

Medically, things were also going well. The group was staying relatively healthy, though some people were hard to convince. Mook had an endless series of minor complaints and needed constant reassurance from me that he wasn't coming apart. I pointed out to him that his pulse was forty beats per minute less than mine and he almost seemed to be putting on weight.

The biggest medical problem so far was my own fault. I made the mistake of casually mentioning that I was taking diamox and maybe that was helping me to do better at Camp II and higher. Some climbers take it routinely, but until this year I hadn't taken it myself. Even though I'm a doctor I have a general philosophical belief that medicines are unnatural and, whenever possible, the body should be given a chance to heal itself without them. This year I concluded that there is nothing natural about being above seventeen thousand feet, so the body doesn't know how to deal with it and needs a little help. Such reasoning allowed me to compromise my principles without feeling guilty.

My casual comment had the effect of causing a run on diamox. Some climbers who didn't routinely take it and who didn't bring any along started asking for it. Having to supply two pills a day to three climbers over two months was seriously depleting my inventory of five hundred pills. Even with the need to maintain an emergency reserve, I figured I would just squeak by until Mook told me he "lost his supply in the tent." Knowing Mook was a smooth salesman, I wasn't sure whether he really lost them, or whether he wanted to double up on his dosage prior to the summit ascent, but feeling fresh from my shower and with the sun still out, I took a walk to the New Zealand camp to see if they had any pills to spare.

There was the usual boisterous scene that I had come to expect and enjoy and even at times to depend upon. Rob was there, as well as Jan and Chantal and a few other climbers, sipping tea and telling jokes. It turned out Jan had plenty of extra diamox. She needed some tetracaine and I offered to supply her with some. Problem solved, I leaned back to enjoy the tea, crackers, and laughter.

Chantal took the chance to tell me, in French, that since I saw her last she had torn a ligament in her knee and was using a brace. I had torn the same ligament years ago and was also using a brace. She asked if I wanted to see hers and I said okay, not realizing she was wearing it. She stood up and pulled her pants down. Eventually, I lowered my eyes to look at her brace. We had been conversing in French and I'm sure everyone else around the table must have wondered just what exactly we had been saying to each other.

I was late getting back to camp and returned in the middle of another meeting. Dave Mencin, a geophysicist familiar with our GPS equipment had hiked into base camp to go over the system with us and to be around for radio consultations in case there was trouble setting up on the summit. He was giving a boring demonstration of how to bolt the stand into the ice. The group was looking for a little relief so I was immediately asked what was going on in the New Zealand camp.

I answered honestly: "Oh, nothing much. Jan and I shared some drugs and Chantal took her pants off."

The meeting droned on until Dave was satisfied everything was working. He was dithering too long with one dial and was losing his audience. A bored climber joked, "I bet I could learn to read that meter in five minutes."

"That's probably about right," Dave answered. "I could teach a yak to do it in two."

When it was finally over, he asked if there were any questions. "Just one," came the reply. "I'd like to ask Ken what color Chantal's underwear is."

Spirits were high. The weather was holding and soon we'd be leaving for the summit. Some climbers filled the time reading and listening to music while others took daily walks in the icefall to not lose their edge. Nima Tashi left for a quick trip to his village of Pangboché to get a blessing from his lama and to buy socks. Everyone prepared in his own way.

At first I firmly believed that I needed rest, but each time someone left for a hike in the icefall I looked on uneasily, fearing that he was gaining some advantage over me. Finally, I gave in to a group invitation to get in some exercise. I didn't have the confidence to resist.

The group had a head start, but as I caught up to them I could see that they had stopped to poke at something with their ice axes. They had come across parts of a skull—a human skull. I recognized the shape of the jaw and the teeth. I didn't have to tell them, though. We all realized it couldn't be anything else. No animal is foolish enough to venture this high.

Someone had gone into the icefall but hadn't made it out the other side. His name, nationality, and date and circumstances of disappearance will have been recorded in the history of Everest, but this area has the highest fatality rate and there would be a lot of possible candidates. We had no idea who the icefall was presenting to us, or why.

Oddly, we didn't talk about it once we left the site. The exercise session was definitely over, though, and we hiked out of the graveyard in silence. I sensed a tacit understanding that this would be something we wouldn't talk about, and try not to even think about, until the expedition was over.

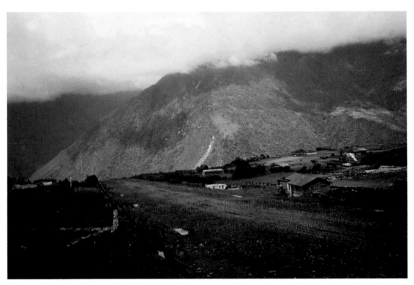

The dirt landing strip in Lukla. A crashed plane lies beside the runway.

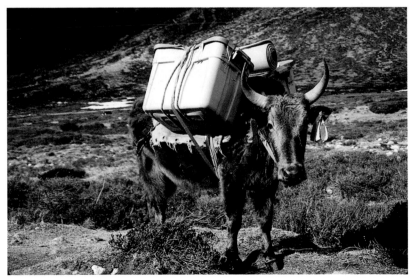

A yak loaded with one of Kamler's four medical supply trunks.

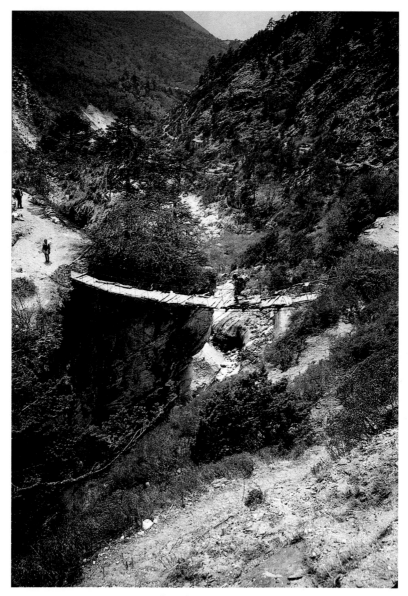

Suspension bridge on route to Everest.

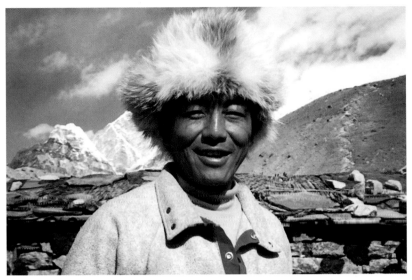

Ong-Chu ready to greet climbers.

(Courtesy FormAsia)

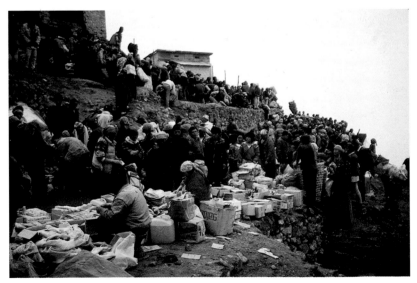

The market at Namché.

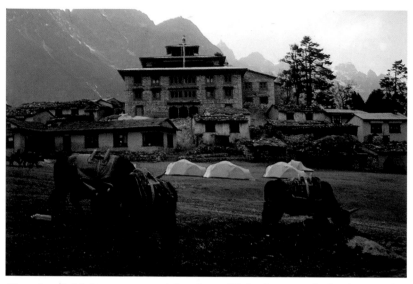

Tangboché Monastery with a handful of tents pitched outside.

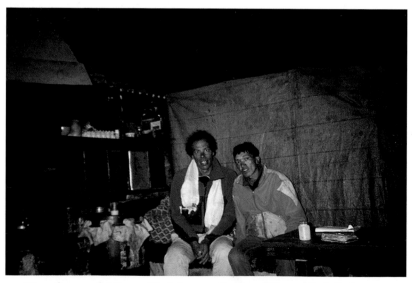

Kamler and Nima Tashi, together at Nima Tashi's home.

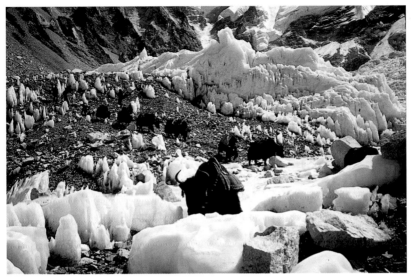

Yaks on the Khumbu Glacier approaching Base Camp.

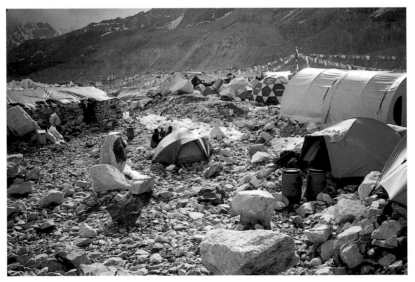

View of Base Camp. The stone hut with the blue tarps to the left is the cook tent. The blue and yellow hexagonal tent is the medical tent. The white dome tent on the right is the mess tent.

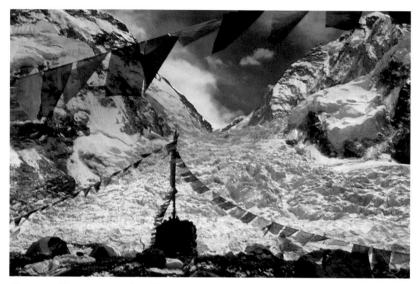

Prayer flags over the lhapso at Base Camp. The icefall is seen in the background.

(Courtesy FormAsia)

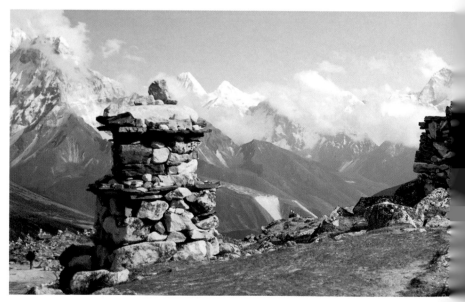

The Sherpa memorial.

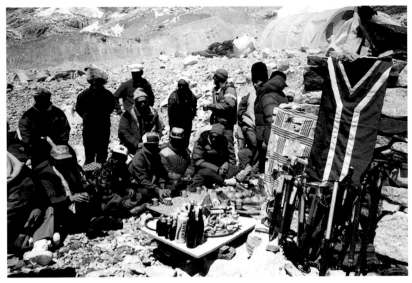

Kamler (kneeling center) with his teammates at the Puja. Offerings are stacked on boards and ice axes are placed at right to be blessed. (Courtesy FormAsia)

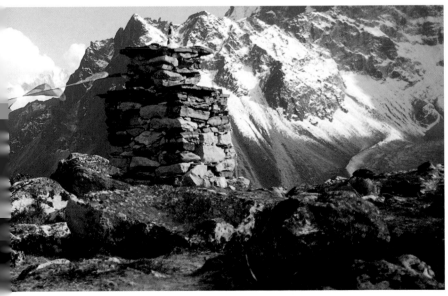

(Courtesy FormAsia)

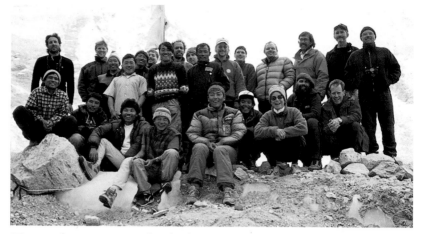

Team photo—1992 climb: (sitting center) Ong-Chu; (kneeling from right) Perry Salmonson, Vern Tejas, Margo Chisholm; (standing 1ˢᵗ and 2ⁿᵈ from left) Pete Athans, Todd Burleson; (standing 6ᵗʰ from left) John Helenick; (standing 8ᵗʰ from left) Kamler; (standing 2ⁿᵈ and 3ʳᵈ from right) Hugh Morton, Skip Horner; (standing 6ᵗʰ from right) Mike Gordon.

(Courtesy Alpine Ascents)

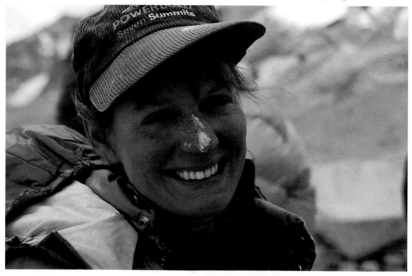

Jan Arnold at Base Camp.

(Courtesy Hall and Ball Archive/Hedaehoa House)

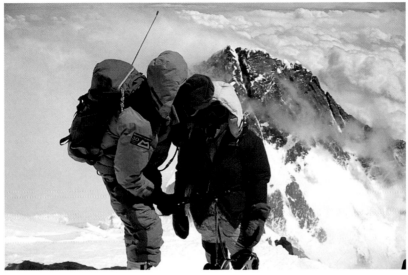

Rob Hall and Chantal Mauduit (in red and yellow) making their way to the summit.

(Courtesy Guy Cotter, Hedgehog House, New Zealand)

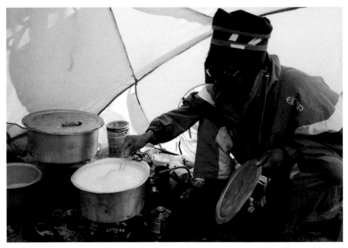

Lakpa-Rita preparing a meal.

(Courtesy FormAsia)

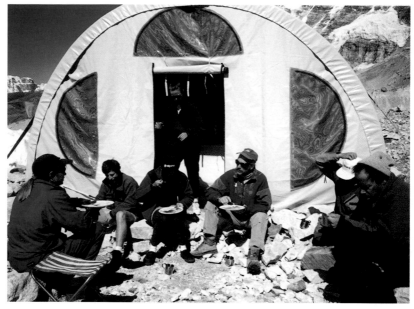

Dining al fresco outside the mess tent. Lily Leonard (left), Jim Williams (right with sunglasses), Kamler (far right).

(Courtesy FormAsia)

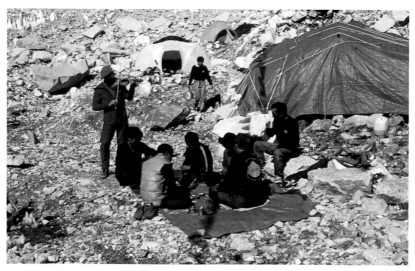

Vern serenading the Sherpas on his violin at Base Camp.

(Courtesy Skip Horner)

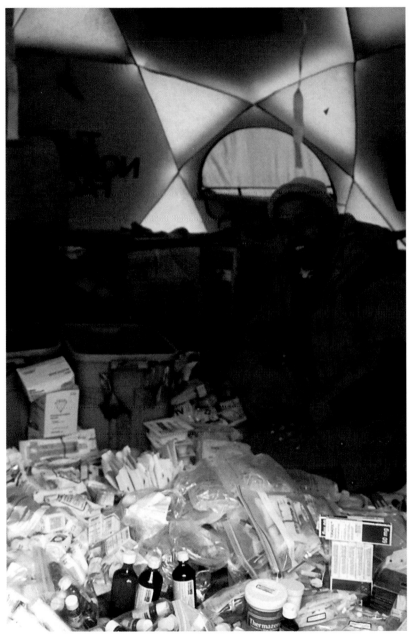

Kamler setting up the medical tent at Base Camp.

(Courtesy FormAsia)

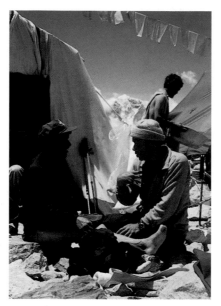

*Kamler at Base Camp splinting
a Sherpa's broken leg.*

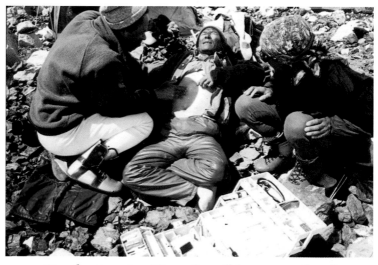

Kamler treating Kima for a "chang overdose."

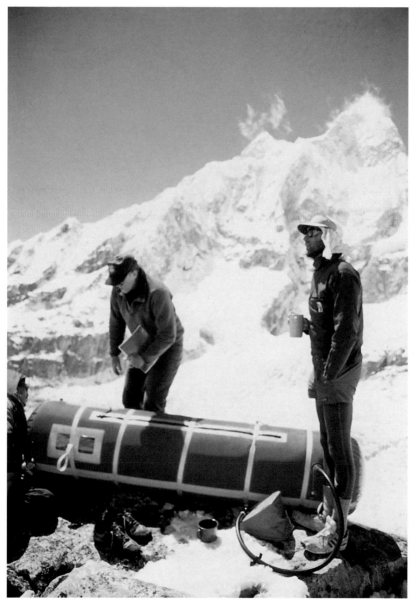

Setting up the Gamoff bag.

(Courtesy Pete Athans)

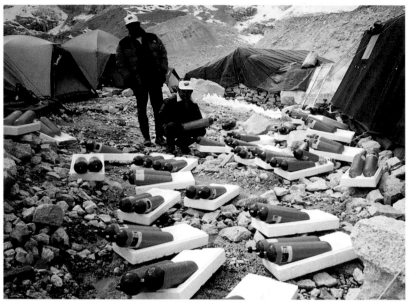

Rob Hall (standing) taking inventory of oxygen tanks.

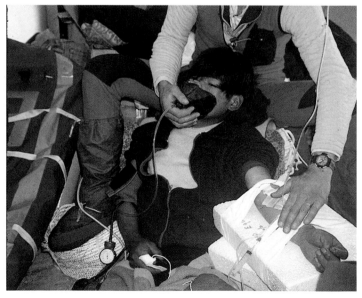

Treating Koncha for pulmonary edema. The Gamoff bag waits ready for use at left.

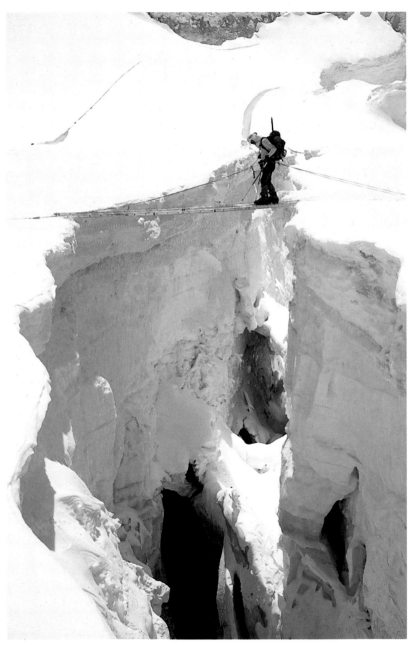

A crevasse can be 10 stories deep or more.

(Courtesy Skip Horner)

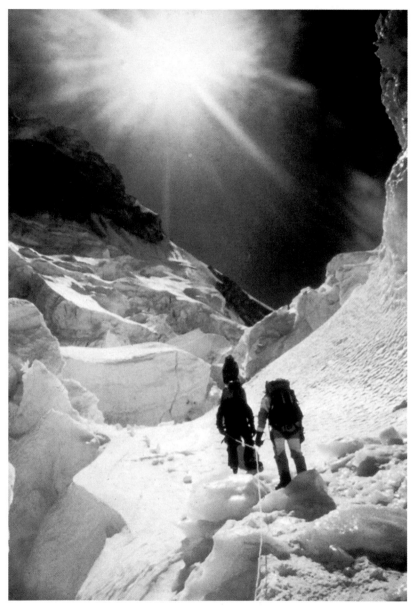

Sunrise over the icefall.

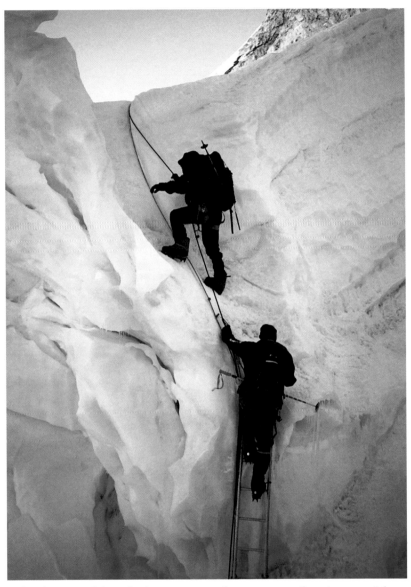

Climbers making their way out of a crevasse that is too wide to cross on ladders. (Courtesy FormAsia)

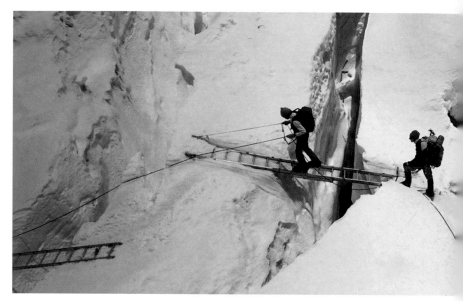

Kamler (in front) crossing a crevasse in the icefall.

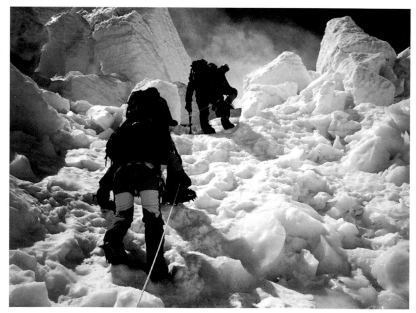

Climbing in the icefall.

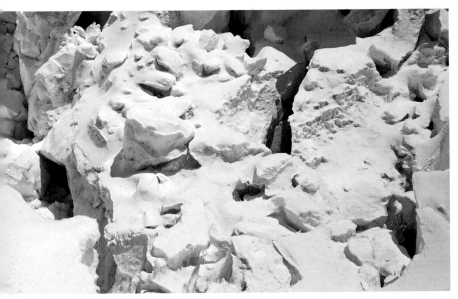

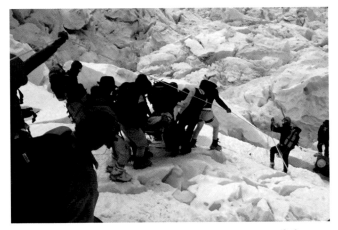

Climbers heroically pulling Pasang-Nuru out of the crevasse.

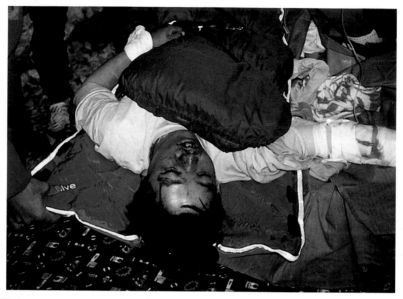

Emergency treatment for Pasang-Nuru after he is rescued from the crevasse.

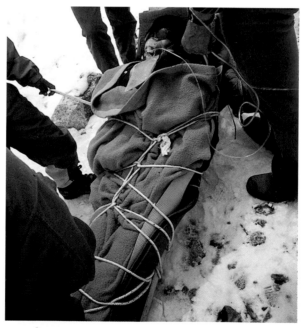

Preparing Pasang-Nuru for evacuation.

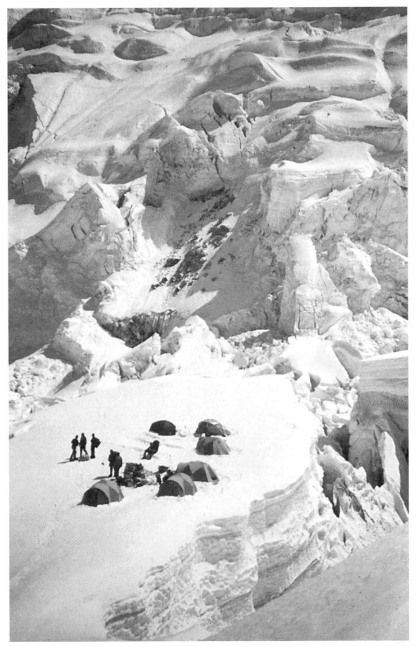

Aerial view of Camp I.

(Courtesy FormAsia)

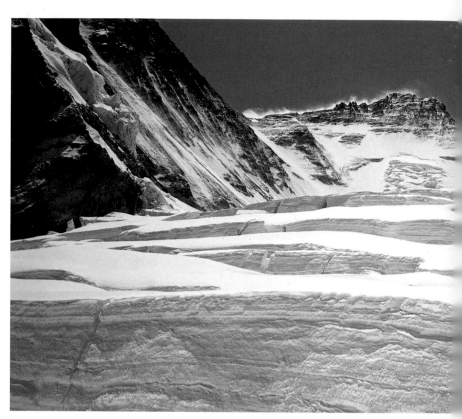

Walking in the Western Cwm.

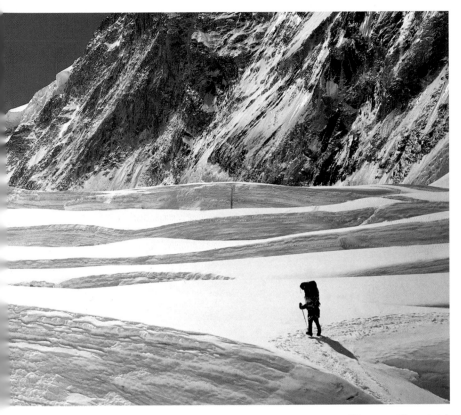

(Courtesy FormAsia)

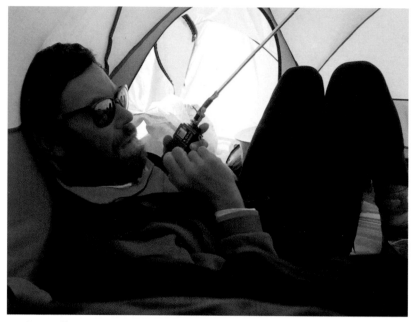

Rob Hall in his tent at Camp III in 1996 holding his radio. Probably the last picture taken of Rob.

(Courtesy FormAsia)

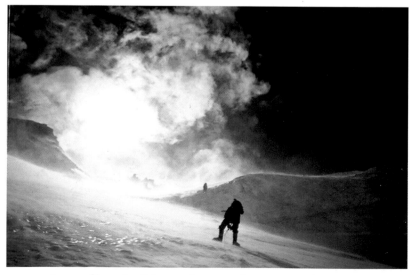

Ascending the Lhotse face on the way to Camp IV.

(Courtesy FormAsia)

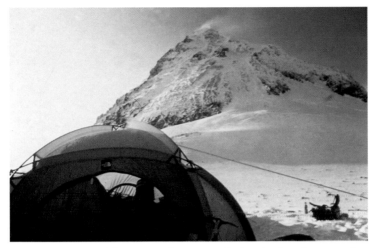

Camp IV with Everest's summit in the background.

(Courtesy FormAsia)

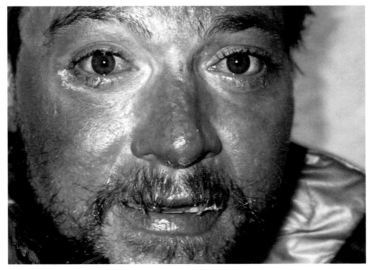

John Helenick, completely snow blind.

(Courtesy FormAsia)

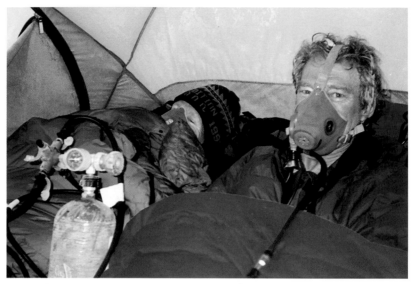

Sleeping on oxygen at Camp IV. Doug Hanson at left.

(Courtesy FormAsia)

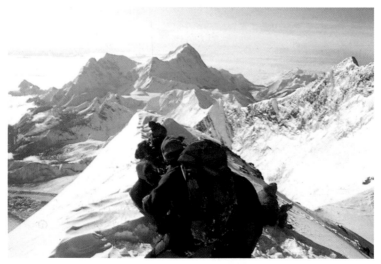

Climbers resting on the Southeast Ridge.

(Courtesy FormAsia)

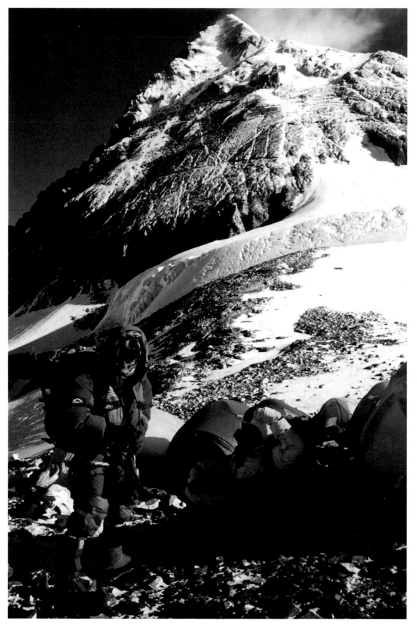

The South Col with Everest's summit in the background.

(Courtesy FormAsia)

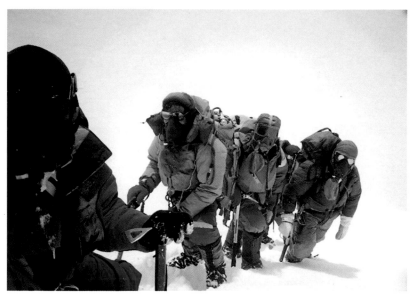

*On oxygen and in deep snow on the Southeast Ridge in 1995.
Kamler is in front.*

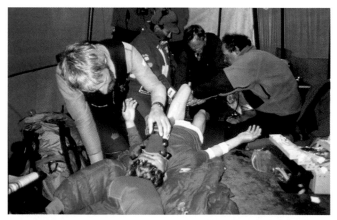

*Kamler (right in green jacket), Heinrick Hansen
(center), Lopsang (at left in green cap) treating
Makalu Gao at Camp II.*

(Courtesy FormAsia)

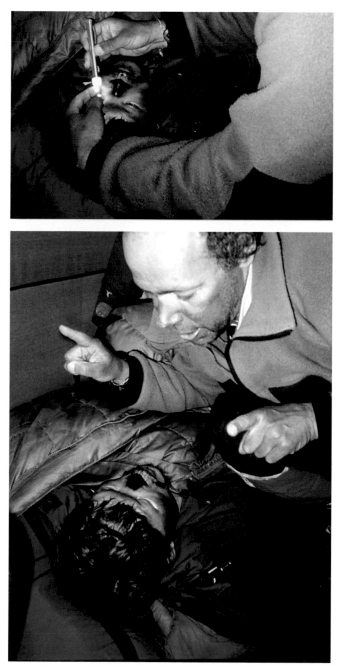

Checking Makalu's eyes for snowblindness.

(Courtesy FormAsia)

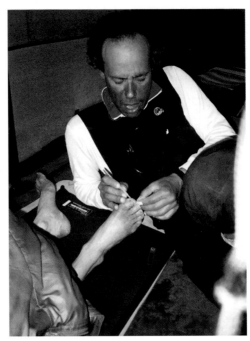

Removing bits of frozen sock from Makalu's toes.

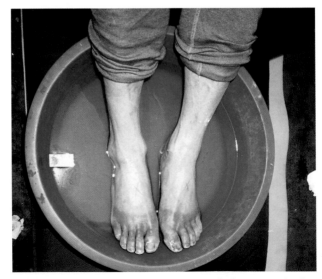

Thawing Makalu's frozen toes. X on each foot marks location of pulse.

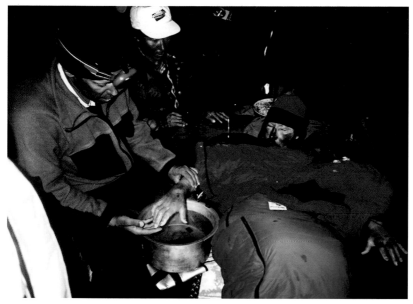

Treating Beck Weathers at Camp II for extreme frostbite.
(Courtesy FormAsia)

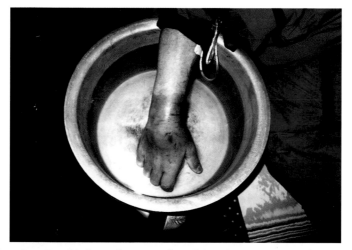

Defrosting Beck's hand. Note the clear demarcation lines of the frostbite.
(Courtesy FormAsia)

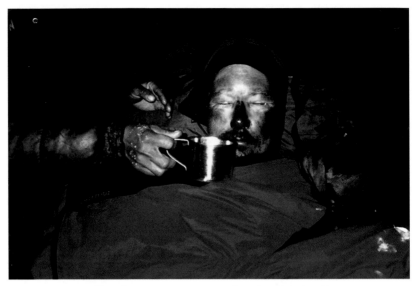

Feeding hot soup to a resting Beck Weathers.

(Courtesy FormAsia)

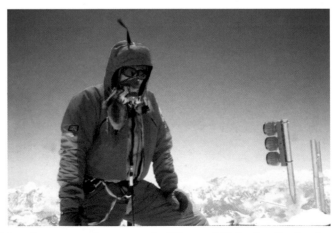

Todd Burleson on the summit. The red light in the background is the GPS laser reflector.

(Courtesy Alpine Ascents)

I was wrong. Teatime came and went with no one mentioning anything, but then just before dinner I overheard one of my secret-sharers tell Todd he had a piece of a human skull in his backpack.

The smile left Todd's face. He said in a low, measured voice, "Don't bring it in the mess tent. Don't show it to any Sherpas. Don't talk about it. Just get it out of camp. It's bad karma."

I thought there wasn't enough smoke coming from the juniper fire that cold morning we started for the summit. I added some fresh branches and Ong-Chu nodded his approval. Once the smoke passed over me I threw a handful of rice at the lhapso and left base camp.

We reached Camp I, all of us tired but in pretty good shape. I thought: One hurdle down. Tomorrow is the Cwm. I'm getting closer to the summit. If I make it I'll never have to climb the icefall again. There's a big difference between wanting to climb Everest and wanting to *have* climbed it. I realized then that I was in the second category.

There is nothing colder than putting on a frozen climbing boot after you've slept all night on ice, except maybe standing around waiting to get going. I timed my routine the next morning to exit the tent the same time as everyone else—not too hard to do considering that except for my boots, I had slept with all my clothes on.

It got even colder when the sun came up and we started off into the wind that had haunted us in our tents all night. It blew unceasingly from the southwest, freezing the left side of my face. I moved up the Cwm wearing a down jacket, balaclava, and three pairs of gloves. With all the bulk, crossing crevasses was dicier than usual, especially when big gusts forced us to maintain our balance in midcrossing by leaning into the wind, out over the side of the ladder. Then, when the wind stopped, we'd suddenly find ourselves teetering over a yawning chasm. Each crevasse too large to cross on ladders was a welcome sight. It meant one less chance to be a weather vane and, since we had to turn to get around it, it meant a brief chance to get the wind off the west side of my face.

Just past the last crevasse was a flat where we usually took a break but it was so cold no one wanted to, except for one climber with diarrhea. I made him take a Lomotil pill on the spot and we continued on. We needed to keep moving to avoid hypothermia, but we also needed liquids to prevent dehydration. We made one quick stop to drink hot water out of our bottles, bundling down against one another like penguins in a roost.

My mouth was frozen by the time I reached Camp II, and I was afraid the hot tea that Dawa and Kami had prepared would crack my teeth. Along with some other Sherpas, they had come up the day before and had a fire going for us in the cook tent. I sipped the tea slowly and felt my mouth defrost.

In the morning, we all felt better. The sun was out, big and bright, and we were having trouble believing we were ever cold. Today would be a rest day. We had to make our final choices on what gear and clothing we'd be taking higher. Extra clothes mean extra weight. The closer you get to the top, the more it pulls you down. On the other hand, to have warm clothes but not have them when you need them is ridiculous, or worse. The memory of yesterday's march was not obscured by today's sunlight.

Todd and Pete held a briefing. The wind had blown most of the snow off the Lhotse Face, exposing the hard blue ice underneath. That meant tougher going; it's much harder to kick steps into ice than into snow. To use our energy efficiently, our crampon points would need to be extra sharp so they'd penetrate the ice easily. Todd also reminded us that, whatever clothes we chose, to avoid hypothermia we must make sure that all zippers lined up so that, when necessary, all the layers could be dropped and raised quickly. This was especially true for Lily, the only female in the group.

Nima Tashi hadn't made it back in time to leave base camp with the team, but he caught up to us at Camp II. I knew he was here because when I went out of my tent to borrow a metal file, I found that my crampons had already been sharpened. I went to thank him and ask if he had gotten the lama's blessing. He said, "Many times." He also had gotten his socks. I supposed we were all set then.

There was a hint of light in the sky when I awoke early the next morning but as the light increased, the air seemed to get colder instead of warmer. I was pleased to not feel any wind as I came outside. The orange glow of the cook tent looked warm and I went directly to it, anxious to not get too chilled. Most of the climbers were there already and Dawa and Kami were earnestly serving up their attempt at porridge. It tasted as awful as usual, but at least I could warm my hands on the side of the bowl.

Once all the climbers had been served, Dawa and Kami took their leave, Kami being careful to leave some extra porridge in a pot in the corner in case anyone wanted more. They joined Pemba and the other climbing Sherpas who were going to Camp III on a roundtrip to drop off supplies. They were anxious to get an early start and left as soon as there was enough light.

We could linger in the tent a little while longer since we would be stopping at III and a later start would give us more light and maybe more warmth.

"Frank, how can you call yourself British?" I asked. "This porridge is an insult to the queen. It tastes like shit."

"I like it when it tastes shitty," he replied.

Secretly I admired a good climber's ability to eat anything. It was a skill I was unable to master.

Leaving our warm confines, we stepped out into the vast cold space outside the tent. In the early light the enormous face of Lhotse took on a blue glow, dominating the scene and our thoughts. This huge mountain would soon be taking our measure. Suddenly there wasn't much talk. We set off like a line of ants, taking microscopic steps and feeling humble and insignificant. I let my mind wander far from the trail. Often a song will come into my head—just one line over and over—and not a song I particularly like. In the company of Buddhist Sherpas I've come to realize that this is my mantra—a phrase of no emotional significance that's chanted continually. It lets the mind drift into a deeper level of consciousness.

It got colder and colder as we crossed the top of the Cwm, jumping over some small crevasses and probing for larger ones with our ski poles. The wind of the past few days had made our work easier by blowing off the superficial snow layer that often covers the crevasses. Despite two layers of gloves, my hands were tingling and I was having trouble controlling my ski poles. I withdrew my fingers into my palms so I could ball them up to decrease heat loss. It helped but it wasn't enough, and my hands soon were numb. We had been moving at a good steady pace, with no complainers, and I hesitated to be the one to break the rhythm but I had to get another pair of gloves on. I called a stop and as I took out my overmitts, almost everyone else reached for more gloves, a scarf, or an extra hat. I saw I wasn't the only one who was cold, nor the only one who didn't want to be the climber who called the stop.

The Western Cwm finishes at the world's most majestic dead end. Ahead of us was Lhotse; to the right, Nuptse; to the left, Everest: three points in a crown of ice over twenty-five thousand feet high. The base of Lhotse bends and cracks where it meets the Cwm. The crack was, for us, a huge moat too big to cross. We detoured around the crevasse, entering Lhotse at its far corner where a snow slope leads up onto the face like an outside ramp.

I was climbing well, I felt strong, and now I wasn't afraid to look up. At the start of the snow slope I tied my ski poles to an anchor. I wouldn't need them anymore. There were no more long flat spots between here and the summit. After a short break, Jim started up the ramp. I followed, with Nima Tashi close behind me. Pete and Wally brought up the rear.

The slope mounted alongside the base of Lhotse and gradually blended into it. We were on a ramp that got narrower and narrower until we were forced against the ice. It ended by diminishing into a ledge and then into just a series of footholds that led onto the sheer face of Lhotse.

Jim stepped out into the footholds, balanced on the front points of his crampons, then clipped into a dangling rope that disappeared over a protruding bulge of blue ice. The rope was the first in a continuous series of anchored lines which led straight up the 45-degree slope to Camp III, fifteen hundred feet above us.

I moved sideways to the end of the ledge, its width now less than the length of my boot. My forward crampons were solidly in the ice but my heels were hanging over the edge. I was waiting for Jim to start up the rope so that I could move into his position. Nima Tashi was on the ledge a step behind me, waiting to move into mine. There was no wind. There was no movement. We were suspended in a quiet moment of anticipation.

Suddenly, above us, there was a rumbling noise but our view was obscured by the overhanging ice bulge. It lasted longer than a second and then a body slid past us, skidding, tumbling, and then bouncing down the slick slope. In sheer horror, we watched as a human being with a face and a hat and a backpack and boots hurtled down the mountain at sickeningly increasing speed, catapulted over the crest of the huge crevasse and landed in the snow out of view on the other side. Jim cried out, "Oh, no; Sherpa, no!" From behind me I heard Lily scream, and then there was silence. Quietly, Nima Tashi said to me he recognized the red hat. It was Kami.

The three of us were on a precarious ledge, but no one moved. Jim radioed to Wally, who was the furthest one back on the slope. Wally hadn't seen what had happened, but while we waited he down-climbed to a position where he could look over the crevasse.

He came back on the radio: "I can see him . . . I don't see any movement." Kami had fallen to the bottom of Lhotse, in an area with hidden crevasses.

We backed down the ledge just far enough so we could stand, and waited while Wally and Pete slowly and carefully, made their way over to where he lay far below us and out of sight. Nobody spoke.

It would be a lot easier for me if he was dead. The selfish, repugnant thought had surfaced immediately and I was ashamed to discover it within me. I couldn't allow it a chance to even fully form in my head so I quickly reburied it by focusing on how to proceed if he was still alive and by adding additional intensity to my hope that somehow he was.

The long silence was broken by Wally's voice on the radio. He said only, "We got to him." Nothing more. Kami's condition was obvious from what Wally didn't say. We all understood.

Slowly we down-climbed from the ledge, being more careful than we had ever been before, until we reached a flat spot at the bottom of the snow slope where we could stop safely. I was the last one down. Tears fell from Lily's eyes and her lower lip was quivering. Frank stood up and embraced me. He was crying too. We held each other a long time until he finally broke away, leaned down over his pack, and hit it. He said, "Why do these things have to happen?" and then hit the pack over and over.

One by one, people regained enough composure to start down. Nima Tashi got up as soon as he saw I was ready. I took a few steps down the slope before he caught up with me and handed me my ski poles. He remembered that I had tied them off on the way up and he had had the presence of mind to get them for me. Maybe I wasn't as composed as I thought.

Nima Tashi slowed his pace to keep me company, though we descended in silence. As we crossed below the giant crevasse, the lower slope came into view and we could see Kami's body at the end of a long streak of blood. Wally and Pete were standing there, unsure if according to Buddhist custom they were allowed to touch the body yet. Dawa joined them. He had raced up from Camp II with my medical kit in the hope that it might be needed, but there was nothing to be done. My job was easy. Recalling that repressed thought, I turned away with a pang of guilt, almost as if I had let him die.

Frank was the only one to not stop and look on the way down, and when I arrived in camp he was sitting on a rock. Each of us picked out a rock as we arrived. None of us was ready to be alone yet.

Behind us there was the slow procession of Wally and Pete and several Sherpas dragging a body bag across the Cwm and into camp. Later, Pete told me that when they got to Kami, they saw that his safety line was still attached to his harness, indicating he hadn't been clipped in. Wally said Kami's limbs were "at crazy angles" and his face was "mush." He used some of my bandages to cover the face before the other Sherpas arrived. "Even so," Wally said, "because we were dragging him there was a lot of leakage through the bag." When they got to camp, they put up a tent and put the body inside. We could smell the incense and hear the prayers.

Pemba and the other Sherpas who had left with Kami this morning returned from their roundtrip and joined us on the rocks. Pemba said that Kami had wanted very much to be a climbing Sherpa and this morning he raced ahead of the others to try to prove himself. He got to Camp III before anyone else and dropped his supply load. As Pemba and the others were still unloading theirs, Kami took off.

"I was just a few minutes behind him," Pemba said. "As I started off I could see the rope all the way down the face. Kami wasn't on it. I knew he must have fallen."

A lot of Sherpas don't clip in to the ropes. It takes time and they always want to show each other how fast they can go. They depend on a "Sherpa rappel"—twisting the rope around their arms and using the friction to hold them back. It's much faster but not very safe. Pemba guessed that Kami had tripped and his hand came free from the rope. Once you start falling on that steep, sheer ice, there is no way to stop. Judging by how soon he didn't see him on the rope, Pemba said he must have slipped right outside the camp.

A conversation ensued:

"He fell two thousand feet then."

"I hope at least he was knocked unconscious right away."

"He wasn't. I heard him scream as he flew by us."

"No, that was me," Lily said.

I mused sadly that Kami had wanted to be the first one down, and he was. This wasn't a tasteless joke, but rather an attempt to use irony to fend off an uncomfortable thought encroaching on me. Frank had asked why these things have to happen and then tried to beat the answer out of his backpack. But the answer wasn't in there. It was with the people who carried the packs. These things happen because we set the scene to make them happen. Once you decide that it's okay to pay people to risk their lives to help you accomplish a frivolous goal, you have to live with the consequences when the odds catch up with them. Kami was young, inexperienced, careless, and he didn't clip in. Todd had said, "At least it was no one else's fault." But it was. It was ours. It always feels better to blame the victim but we were responsible for Kami's death. Enticing these people to risk their lives for us is an abuse of power. We exploit them in the name of sport, offering them easy money and expedition glamour, and they don't stand a chance.

Yet it would be a mistake to blame ourselves entirely and not recognize that Kami's motivation had to be internal as well. He was responding to a deeply felt need to prove himself, impress others, taste glory, or whatever else it is that brings people to the highest mountains. In that way, he was no different than us. We had merely given him the opportunity to test himself—and to kill himself.

The rock I was sitting on was getting harder. I went to the cook tent for a cup of tea and some subdued lighting. The pot of porridge was still there that Kami had thoughtfully left in case anyone wanted seconds. Now I felt bad for not liking it this morning.

There are no set customs, no standard rules on whether a climb should be continued after a death. A decision can't be made until it happens because the effect on the expedition is the sum of the impact on each member. None of us had a sustained feeling to cancel the expedition. Nothing even as formal as a consensus was needed. There was just a shared understanding that we would continue. You can honestly consider people of all cultures to be equal, but it would be a lie to pretend you identify with them all equally.

A young man cut down at the beginning of his potential is a universally understood tragedy. Our grief was real but the impact wasn't the same as it would have been were he "one of us."

A realistic and uncomfortable thought was easily avoided by invoking science. The GPS still needed to be put up and that was enough justification for being here and continuing on, though no one would deny that if it didn't have to be carried to the summit, we'd be a lot less interested in the project. We were here for the method, not the goal, but the GPS conveniently made it unnecessary to examine other motives which could prove selfish or egotistical.

In the morning, rows of prayer flags were strung up over the camp, a vibrant display in the early sunlight. The funeral procession, led by Todd and Lakpa-Rita, crossed under the colorful canopy, starting on its laborious way down the Cwm and the icefall. With the bright, cloudless sky, it was probably the nicest day since we'd been at Camp II.

Lakpa-Rita was crying when he left. He had taken Kami from his own tiny village of Tamé and had reassured his mother that he would take good care of her only son. Now he was bringing him back for cremation.

Todd felt strongly that as expedition leader, he had to go too. The descent would take three or four days. Then there were the ceremonies, after which he felt that out of respect he would need to stay a day or two before he could take his leave. But if we were to make another summit attempt, we'd have to start within the next few days. Our supplies wouldn't last much longer and the weather window would be closing. Todd knew as he left the camp that he was marching right out of the expedition.

The absence of Kami was obvious and painful as Dawa served us breakfast without his tentmate and assistant. Other climbers stopped by in the way one would expect when there was a death in the family, offering "condolences on the loss of your Sherpa."

Dawa was asked how he was managing. He said the cooking was okay but he had to change tents. "In my tent last night," he said, "there was too much imagination."

We took advantage of the rare afternoon sunlight to sit outside, watching Nima Tashi coil the same rope three times and listening to radio reports from the New Zealand expedition. We were delayed, to say the least, but Rob's team, after also having spent a night here, had continued on up and today had been their summit day. It was perfectly calm for us at Camp II and Radio Nepal's weather report was for "a pleasant day throughout the kingdom," but the Kiwis, five thousand feet above us, had been beaten back after they encountered high winds and deep snow. Everest is full of surprises—most of them bad ones.

The Kiwis, unable to summit, straggled in to Camp II the following day, still in full retreat. Rob stopped by my tent to tell me they had had "a bit of a hard go." With Jan down at base camp, I thought the team would appreciate a house call.

They did. Rob was most concerned about Chantal, who had been carried part of the way down, complaining of pain in her chest. The drop in altitude had revived her, though, and by the time I saw her, she was full of energy and her usual self. Her lungs were clear. The pain was between her ribs and felt to me like a small tear in the intercostal muscles that expand the ribs for deep breathing—no surprise since Chantal had been climbing without oxygen.

After confirming that Chantal was okay, I made rounds of all the other climbers. Guy Cotter, Rob's guide, had some frostbitten toes and was exhausted from bringing down Chantal and helping with another climber, Doug Hansen. A postal worker from Seattle, Doug was an experienced mountaineer, yet he had descended part of the route below the South Summit without clipping into the fixed line. Just a few days ago we had seen what a fatal error that could be, but it's hard to think clearly when you're that high on Everest.

When I entered Doug's tent he was putting in eye drops to treat a mild case of snow blindness. They were the drops I had given Jan the day we traded drugs at base camp. He wanted me to check his frostbitten toes, and as I examined them he spoke wistfully about how close he had come to the summit. The toes were frightful—red, swollen and blistered—but, I reassured him, those were all signs that they'd recover fully. There wasn't enough damage to prevent him from climbing again nor, as it turned out, enough to prevent him from his fateful return to Everest the following year.

It seemed to us the Kiwis had pushed too hard—staying out above twenty-six thousand feet for over twenty hours, then having to stumble back in the dark. They had cut their safety margin close and though there were no serious injuries, perhaps Rob was getting too familiar with the mountain.

The Kiwis would be heading down in the morning and that would leave no other team on the mountain except us. Though they hadn't summited, Rob remained in good cheer and was as selfless as ever. He loved being in the mountains and wanted to see a successful climb even if it wasn't his. He told us in detail what conditions were like above Camp IV, where they had run into trouble and where he and his lead Sherpa, Lopsang, had left fixed ropes and anchors that might help us. He wished us luck and said, "The mountain is all yours."

Fast-moving cirrus clouds were shredding as they collided with the top of Lhotse. You didn't have to be a weatherman to know it was cold and windy up there. Maybe our weather window was closing. We discussed the possibility over a light lunch. For the past two days, all our meals had been "light"—we were running out of food. Reluctantly we agreed that we would gear up in the morning and make a move. We either had to go up or go down.

Wally came into the mess tent while we were having breakfast and said optimistically, "The weather looks great." But Wally is always optimistic; It was four-thirty in the morning and still completely dark out. The stars were turning off and on in clusters and as it got light we could see the high, windswept clouds that had been intermittently obscuring those stars.

"The wind seems to be moving away," Jim said, adding his own note of optimism. "It's pushing the clouds over the summit and into Tibet." He half believed it and half hoped that saying it would make it so.

No one wanted to go down, but no one was ready to be foolish either. We agreed that we would don full battle array and head off across the Cwm one more time, delaying our final decision until we reached the fixed ropes. We wouldn't start up unless the clouds slowed down.

Dangling like a lure, the first fixed rope was in full view before us. After three hours the weather was still marginal so before we took the bait, we needed to make a decision. Camp III is a nowhere, unpleasant place—just a notch chopped in the ice halfway up the Lhotse Face. If we went to III it was with the idea that the next morning we'd start on oxygen, move right up to IV and then, after a short rest, go for the summit. From here on, there was no time, and no place, to call time-out to wait for the weather.

"The clouds have gone to Tibet . . . and they weren't ripped up by the summit." Jim's observation was enough to tip the balance since climbers would rather go up than down anyway. One by one on cue, we moved out onto the ledge, beginning the elaborate choreography of a summit launch.

Poised with my feet over the edge and my carabiner hooked into the rope, I was in precisely the position I had been in three days ago, looking up at the same ice bulge. I paused, as I had then, but held it an extra beat as if to be sure that this time, no human meteor would be coming down from above.

The rope to which I was attached ran, in connected segments, straight up the mountain at a relentless 45-degree angle. I slid my jumar (a gripper which locks on the rope when pulled down) an arm's length up the rope until its tether was taut enough against my harness to take my weight as I leaned back. With my legs no longer holding me up, I was free to step up against the side of the ice bulge, kicking my crampon points into the hard ice. Pulling up on the rope brought me upright again, ready to advance the jumar and begin the sequence once more. I was now one step above the ledge—my first in a slow motion walk up the four-thousand-foot face of Lhotse.

The worst parts were at the beginning and at the end. The ice bulge projected out from the face, steepening the climbing angle to 60 degrees. After the first three pitches (section of a climb equal to the length of the rope), I surmounted the bulge and the angle receded to 45 degrees. More snow sticks to the slope at that angle, making it a little easier to kick footholds, but they still have to be done one by one. Kick into the ice, step up on the crampons, slide the jumar higher, start again. The repetition was broken at the top of each pitch where the rope was attached to an anchoring screw embedded in the ice. Switching to the next higher rope requires detaching your carabiner from the rope you're on but not before you've attached another carabiner to the one above, otherwise you have nothing but crampon points holding you against the slope. It's a simple two-step sequence—easy to remember unless your brain has been dulled by endless repetition, fatigue, and lack of oxygen.

Pitch after pitch after endless pitch, higher and slower. Although each anchoring point was a milestone, I came to dread its arrival at the end of a rope. It meant clearing away the monotony that overtook me during each pitch, then bending over to make the switch while breathing with a compressed diaphragm. It routinely took me longer to catch my breath after that maneuver than it did after climbing the pitch that led up to it.

There was no place to rest other than on my feet. When my lungs fell too far behind in filling my oxygen demands, I simply leaned back, perpendicular to the slope, and let the jumar take my full weight. I focused on the intricate details of the ice in front of me while my lungs caught up. It's an effective way to relax as long as you are able to not think about where you are.

Higher and higher and slower and slower. To my left I saw I was drawing even with "the rock"—the only exposed piece of rock on the entire Lhotse Face. It was visible from Camp II to the side of and just below Camp III. If I was approaching that level now, I was making good progress, but the going was getting tougher. The slope steepened quite a bit with a lot more exposed hard ice. As I moved through it I realized this must be the "hard part" just before Camp III. Looking out at my reference rock on the face, I saw that I was now above it. The camp had to be close. Sure enough, two more hard pitches and I could see the yellow tent cloth. Once it was in sight I gave in to my body's urge to relax, holding back just enough energy to reach the tents. But what I reached were rags—shredded tents from a previous expedition. Our tents were higher. Having foolishly allowed my energy reserve to dissipate, I was now unable to call it back. I was on empty. I finished the climb on fumes.

Camp III was three small tents improbably stuck against the side of Lhotse—poor accommodations for the fourth highest mountain in the world. But then, the gods who live here have no reason to provide space to intruders. The best we can hope for is that for a short while they will tolerate our presence. At this altitude there isn't much oxygen but there is a lot of Buddhism in the air.

Lhotse's face is smooth. She has no wrinkles big enough for a tent. At a random spot about halfway up, Sherpas had chopped down into the slope, removed a wedge of ice and then squared off the bottom to form a step. The upslope was undercut and the downslope was reinforced with ice blocks to make a platform just big enough for the tents. Ice screws at the bottom held the tents down; ropes at the top, which attached to ice screws in the back wall, kept the tents from falling forward.

This was no place to go for a stroll. Hard against the back of the tent was the ice slope. Looking out the back door had the same claustrophobic effect as opening a city apartment window that faces the wall of another building. But out the front door of our perch there was an immediate and spectacular two-thousand-foot drop to the Cwm.

Cooking had to be done inside one of the tents. Our chef for the evening, formerly known as Pete, was renamed Pierre in the hope it would make the food taste better. Chef Pierre's specialty was melting snow, which he did by hanging a burner from a carabiner hooked into the tent frame and then putting a pot over it. As fast as the snow melted, we used it to make hot drinks and boil the food packets which had frozen solidly while stored in the camp.

To conserve our strength, stay warm, and rest well, we slept on oxygen, lying alongside the tanks with masks on our faces. I had a dream for the first time since I'd been on the mountain. I guess some higher cerebral functions like dreaming don't occur unless there is a lot of oxygen in the brain.

The dream was vivid: I was at home resting up before going back to Everest for the summit push. The house was warm and the kids were in pajamas sleeping on the floor. Josiane was wearing a heavy white wool sweater and my head was tucked softly against her chest. She started to take the sweater off but I didn't let her, afraid she would get cold. I woke up feeling relaxed and refreshed. The oxygen had made a big difference. It had given me a chance to go home.

As if a switch had been flipped, the tent became illuminated by a brilliant morning sun and within a few minutes the temperature went from too cold to too hot. Outside, in the clear sky, there were puffy clouds drifting slowly over Everest. The wind had broken. All we needed now were two calm days and we could be on top. Though many people have made it this far and not summited, climbing Everest suddenly seemed possible and I allowed myself to get excited at the idea.

Lhotse part two was like Lhotse part one, only higher. We were above twenty-four thousand feet now and the rest of the climb would be on oxygen. I was breathing through a face mask which covered my nose and mouth and was connected by a rubber tube to a regulator on one of two oxygen bottles in my backpack. The fixed ropes continued to draw us straight up at the same boring angle over packed snow mixed with patches of ice. The Sherpas climbing with us were each carrying double loads, trying to make up for the others who were still down in Tamé with Lakpa-Rita and Todd. Despite the extra weight, and because of it, they all moved on ahead of us, anxious to reach Camp IV and get rid of their loads. All except Nima Tashi who wanted to stay with me, bearing his burden at a painfully slow speed.

High up on the mountain the route turned sharply left. The Lhotse Face has to be traversed from one side to the other to get onto the final approach to Everest. The fixed lines now ran directly across the slope. The snow was loose and often gave way under foot. A slip here would bowstring the rope between two anchor points and leave you dangling from the middle, hanging by your carabiner. It wouldn't be fatal but would, at the least, be embarrassing.

The traverse goes over the Yellow Band, an outcropping of yellow-brown rock that rises abruptly out of the ice. It's a tricky crossing because with crampons on, you can't grip the rock. Still, I scratched across it with no slips and no embarrassing moments.

At the end of the traverse is the Geneva Spur, a mass of rock and snow great enough to be a mountain itself. I was about to start up it when Nima Tashi called to me to wait. He calculated that I'd be low on oxygen about now and thought this would be a good place to switch tanks, before the route became steep again. He made the change for me so I wouldn't have to take my pack off but then we both heard a hiss in the line. Afraid it was a leak, we fooled around with the equipment a long time before deciding that either it wasn't a leak or there was nothing we could do about it.

As I climbed higher up the spur, there was less ambient air and the oxygen coming through the tube didn't seem to be adequate. The mask felt claustrophobic. Every time I made a hard move I had to hold it open at the bottom to let more outside air in. When I saw something difficult coming up, I would breathe hard in advance, preloading to get a headstart.

At the top of the spur there was a sudden spectacular view of Everest, up close and huge, right in front of me. The size of it was shocking and it was only the top part—the last three thousand feet that I would have to climb tomorrow.

Camp IV was slightly below me, and after a gentle descent I walked onto the South Col, twenty-six thousand feet up. It was a rubbly rock-and-ice saddle dominated by the looming presence of Lhotse on one side and Everest on the other. The camp was a small cluster of orange tents surrounded by a field of empty oxygen bottles left behind by climbers anxious to descend with as little extra weight as possible. Camp IV was an open, more agreeable place than Camp III but much higher, colder, and windier. Seeing how broad, flat, and featureless the Col was, would make it easy for me next year to visualize those climbers who got lost up here during the storm. Now, though, as we arrived, the sun was still out and there was hardly any wind. We were at the last stop before the summit.

Nima Tashi and I sat down on some empty oxygen bottles. We fiddled some more with my regulator but couldn't find anything wrong. I began to suspect the hiss was normal and my difficulties with the mask were brought on by nervousness combined with the power of suggestion. Maybe Nima Tashi had concluded the same thing but didn't want to tell me.

He did confide in me momentarily that his ankle was sore, but when I asked him more about it he said, "No, no, it's okay." I didn't know how it could not be sore. He has no ankle. I had told him he'd never be able to climb again but now here we were, side by side, one day below the summit of Mount Everest.

Assuming the weather held, we'd leave at midnight, only six hours away. Climbing Everest seemed very possible now and I even dared to imagine myself on the summit. Our excited chatter rapidly subsided as we each found a sleeping bag and an oxygen tank and tried to relax. The camp became eerily quiet.

I was too excited to sleep but too tired to stay awake. I drifted into a quasi-sleep state and, with the oxygen mask on my face, imagined I was under anesthesia. Pete poked me once and I was fully awake again.It was easier to get up at eleven o'clock in the evening than it would have been to get up, after much more sleep, at four o'clock in the morning (our usual starting time for the icefall). In the early morning the body is physiologically at its lowest ebb and it's the hardest time to get going. It's the reason why surprise attacks are often carried out just before dawn.

Someone outside the tent asked if I wanted onion soup. Forgetting where I was for the moment, I stupidly said no, thinking there would be another choice. All I had was hot water and crackers, which I ate while staring at the thermometer in our tiny two-man tent. Although there were three of us huddled inside, the temperature read 30 degrees below zero.

I had to come out of the tent to put on my equipment. The air was still and very cold. The sky was black except for a sharp silver moon, two-thirds full. It provided enough light to cast a deep blue glow on the ice fields. Although I could see well enough to put on my harness and crampons and then load two oxygen cylinders in my backpack, I had to switch on my headlight to be sure the gauges read full. Each cylinder weighed seven pounds, but other than that, I was carrying very little—a few chocolate bars, an extra pair of gloves, and three dolls. I tucked a bottle of hot water inside my jacket so it would stay warm.

The expedition became a string of lights—each climber a yellow dot against the deep blue background. Unroped, but in a line, we walked across the Col directly into a broad snow gully called the triangular face. The first headlight was Pete, our strongest climber. I was toward the rear, just ahead of Nima Tashi and Jim. It's important to keep some really strong people at the back (Nima Tashi and Jim, not me) in case there's a problem. The gully began gradually but quickly steepened. Our line of lights became more vertical and the spacing less even, as each climber progressed at his own rate. There was no wind to break the silence of the night, just the methodical clinking of ice tools and occasional quiet talk. Voices took on an odd hushed quality, the sound being quickly lost in the vast stillness around us.

The headlight in front of me came steadily closer. It belonged to one of our usually strong climbers, but he seemed to be losing power early on as we worked our way through powdery snow. The snow was too loose to form steps, so as the slope steepened, we relied more and more on our hands. Ahead was a fixed rope. Rob's team had encountered the same problem with traction and put in the rope when they were here a few days ago. It showed up just where he said it would be. Once we started up the rope, the light ahead of me slowed and slowed, then finally stopped. My light soon illuminated the back of a down jacket and the cause of the climber's exhaustion. He was overdressed. He had been working strenuously enough to overheat despite an outside temperature of at least 30 degrees below zero.

He was in an impossible place to pass. Nima Tashi came up behind me, then Jim. The snow around us was too soft to push up against—our feet just slipped right through. Jim coaxed the climber to a spot a little higher up where the snow was slightly harder. It still couldn't take our full weight, but with him hanging off to one side I was able to place a jumar above him and pull myself up hand over hand. Nima Tashi did the same and we continued up, leaving Jim behind to help the climber undress.

The line of lights was now pretty far above me, and as I climbed, each light disappeared one by one. That meant the slope crested and flattened out on the other side, at least enough to block the lights from my line of sight. The crest turned out to be a rock buttress, and when I finally got over it I was relieved to see that the others weren't too far ahead. I expected I'd be up with them in a few more minutes but then immediately realized why they hadn't progressed further; I plunged into much deeper, drier snow. There were no discernible footprints ahead of me, just a trough where legs had waded into powder too loose to take a shape.

The line of lights was taking on a more random appearance as everyone, including the Sherpas, was getting tired and stopping individually for short breaks. I passed Frank who had sat down in the snow (or collapsed, it was hard to tell which) for a few minutes' rest.

"Ken, I'm out of oxygen. Could Nima Tashi change tanks for me?"

"Sure, just ask him when he comes up."

"No, it has to come from you." So I waited with Frank a few minutes for Nima Tashi to catch up. I was too tired to change his tank myself. Nima stopped right away to help and then told me I was almost out of oxygen too. Our regulators were continuous flow, not demand flow, so if they were set at the same rate, everyone would run out at about the same time. Wanting to make use of every bit of oxygen, I told Nima I'd continue up another twenty yards or so to a small outcropping of rock which made a flat spot. Mook and Lily were already on it, helping each other change tanks as I approached.

Suddenly my body weight doubled and I was being pulled down into the snow. I could still see Mook and Lily but not the rock they were on. It was obscured by a ring of tingling lights. The scene around me became surreal, like I wasn't part of it anymore. But my reasoning remained intact; I knew I was out of oxygen.

Nima Tashi was right behind me to unscrew my regulator and connect it to the second tank. My head cleared up instantly, my peripheral vision returned, and strength flowed back into my legs. Oxygen was a wonder drug.

For some time the sky had been growing brighter and now I was getting uneasy—it was too light. The plan was to reach the southeast ridge at sunrise. We could climb the triangular face in the dark but the ridge required daylight. Getting there too soon would mean waiting around for the light but getting there too late meant lost climbing time. We were behind schedule and I didn't want to see the sunrise yet, but there it was. I looked at the ridge. It wasn't very far away but we were going to be an hour late.

The ridge was overpoweringly spectacular. As I came up on it the world opened below me. Standing on a minuscule edge eight feet wide I was surrounded by an incomprehensibly vast emptiness. I had climbed into outer space, far enough above the planet to look down on immense ice-covered mountains and to see the curvature of the earth. The scene was too unreal to be scary. I was on a stage and the mountains below me were nothing more than a painted backdrop.

With all the climbers collected close together it seemed to be an almost intimate setting. We were sitting in a line along a piece of the edge that we imagined to be slightly flatter than the rest. Sitting was a little tricky because the loose snow didn't really hold and leaning back wouldn't be a good idea. Nevertheless this was our first break and I relaxed in front of the breathtaking panorama, though most of my breath had already been taken.

I didn't need confirmation that we weren't progressing well, but Pete's demeanor and the look on his face confirmed it anyway. We were tired, especially the Sherpas. The extra loads they had carried took their toll and they didn't have the reserve strength to deal with unexpectedly deep snow. We had used more oxygen than we should have to get this far. Tanks should have been changed on the ridge, not before. Being one hour behind wouldn't mean much if it were due to a single event like an equipment problem, since we had a few hours of safety margin built into the schedule. But the delay was due to slow progress which was likely to continue. Ahead up the ridge toward the South Summit, the snow looked the same as what we had been wading through all night. The feeling that we weren't going to make it was in everybody's mind, though no one said it. Pete told us to turn our flow rate down to one and a half liters per minute (we had been going at two) to conserve oxygen. I hated to hear that because it just about doomed the expedition. With less oxygen we'd be moving even slower, but we had no choice. It would be far worse, and maybe fatal, to charge ahead and then suddenly run out of oxygen at an even higher altitude.

The summit was fifteen hundred vertical feet above us, along a crooked seam tilting 15 degrees from left to right and angling 30 degrees upward. The edge was the top of a triangle formed by the junction of the massive southwest face and the even more massive east face. To the left was an eight-thousand-foot drop into Nepal. To the right, a twelve-thousand-foot drop into Tibet. With Pete and Dorgi, our strongest Sherpa, in the lead, we stepped along the edge in single file and unroped. A slip here would start a freefall down the mountain, impossible for another climber to arrest. There was no point in connecting a rope to jerk someone else off the edge. One would be more than enough.

Conditions changed, but not in the way we had hoped. The snow got deeper. At the start of the ridge it was knee high but soon we were plowing forward with our bodies through waist-high snow, not even able to see our boots as we pushed them forward, swinging from one hip and then the other. The snow was reluctant to part before us but was so dry and granular that it immediately collapsed back around us, leaving almost no trace that we had passed through. Each person was breaking his own trail.

I was walking a crooked line without being quite sure where my feet were since I couldn't see them. With each step I tried to feel firmly packed snow with my crampon before putting weight down on my boot. Slowly and carefully we continued up toward the South Summit. The weather was holding. It was a clear, cold day without much wind to blow the snow around. Visibility was good except for occasional periods of "fog," which at twenty-eight thousand feet were actually clouds we passed through. At times I stopped to wait for them to go by because I couldn't be sure if I was about to put my foot down on snow or in a cloud.

After two hours of tentative, measured steps, we had made very little progress. Even more discouraging, Pete and Dorgi, still in the lead, were now making even less. The slope was increasing and the new angle was proving to be too much to surmount on the ball bearings of snow that had been thrown in our path. After they had each taken a few turns stepping up and sliding down, Pete lay against the slope while Dorgi climbed on him to put in an ice screw as high up as he could. Pete fed him a rope but before they could even test it, it pulled out. They were climbing in a bowl of sugar.

We were at 28,100 feet—the buttress of the South Summit, a prominence in the ridge after which the angle lessens the rest of the way. The summit was only nine hundred feet higher. It had taken us two months to get here and with normal snow conditions, it would only take two more hours to reach the top.

But we were in snow that was now chest high. Although it was only noon, we would need at least another four or five hours to reach the top. That would mean coming back down in the dark, exhausted and on very low (or more likely, no) oxygen. It was obvious Everest didn't want us on the summit.

It was time to talk but we were strung out along the ridge and there was no place to collect. We clumped together in three bunches over our three radios. The decision to turn around was immediate and unanimous but we talked about it a while anyway, restating the obvious again and again. We needed some time to turn ourselves around mentally before starting on a long, disappointing and dangerous descent.

I thought about the last group to be up on this ridge a few days ago. Rob's team had continued on for nearly too long and the condition they returned in confirmed that they had pushed the limits. Our calculations of climbing speed, oxygen consumption, and remaining daylight indicated we should turn around now while we still had an adequate safety margin. But disappointed climbers descending a treacherous ridge is a combination that can easily end in disaster. Climbing accidents are eight times more common on the way down. The memory of Kami's fall was still vivid in my mind. This wasn't over yet. I needed all my concentration now to get down safely, with no more surprises.

Looking back instead of up for the first time, I realized how precarious our position was. We had to descend this same ridge covered with loose, slippery snow that was now sloping 30 degrees downward. Because of the danger of falling forward, I backed down the slope, looking between my legs to see where to place my feet. By digging in my ice ax and holding it with both hands, I anchored myself, then stepped out and down. Only after both boots were on something solid did I remove the ax to reposition it. For the few seconds it took to dig it in lower down I was dependent on my footholds, which never felt really solid. Several times I stopped a slide by jamming the ax back in quickly.

Breathing heavily, with my head bent down, warm oxygen and water vapor accumulated rapidly in my face mask. It fogged my goggles, but I only stopped to wipe them when I couldn't see at all. As long as I had at least one corner of vision I kept going, repeating the same maneuvers over and over and over, patiently resisting an increasing temptation to take life-threatening shortcuts.

That spot at the start of the ridge where we had taken our break on the way up seemed a lot more comfortable on the way down—especially since there were oxygen tanks stashed here. After we left for the summit, a second team of support Sherpas left Camp IV to deposit extra oxygen where we calculated we'd be when the supply we were carrying ran out. That way we each had a third tank for the rest of the descent. Our Sherpas were careful to pick up the empties, as they were supposed to do to keep the mountain clean. Instead of loading them in their packs though, they tossed them into Tibet. They didn't have the strength to carry them down and they didn't want to leave any traces.

The triangular face is not exposed like the ridge and the first part is not as steep—conditions that sometimes work for a glissade, an energy-saving technique of sliding down the mountain on your butt, steering and breaking with your ice ax. Everyone thought the snow was too soft but I was tired enough to try it. Everyone was right. I sank in the snow but discovered that by paddling my feet I could move like a pedal boat. Though I knew everyone above would be laughing, the technique worked and I slid a long way until the slope steepened again. It would be too quick a ride down the face if the snow stopped holding me back so I changed again into a pedestrian. Looking up to see how far I'd come, I saw to my surprise that everyone—everyone—was coming down the same way I had. The slope looked like an amusement park ride.

A long tiring descent still remained, all the more tedious because we hadn't summited. Nearly everyone passed me sooner or later, but they weren't faster, just less slow. Loyalty kept Nima Tashi behind me the whole way. Dorgi was so exhausted that I actually went ahead of him. Passing a Sherpa was a mountaineering first for me.

Lying outside my tent at Camp IV, I was too tired to be disappointed. The night would be cold, there was hardly any food or liquid around and I was dehydrated. We had been over twenty-six thousand feet for sixteen hours. We had reached the South Summit and at that moment were the highest people on earth. I took out my water bottle to enjoy the last few sips. Instead, I got a reminder of how thin the margin is between life and death at this altitude. The water, which I had been carrying inside my jacket, against my chest, was frozen solid.

"How do you feel?" Wally asked me in the morning.

"Okay."

"That's funny, because you look terrible. Your face is peeling and your eyes are bloodshot. I came by to take your photo so we have a record of how bad you look in case you get better."

I obliged him, especially since he offered me hot tea as well.

He continued. "It got a little dicey up there yesterday, didn't it?"

"Yeah," I replied. "A couple of times I started to lose my balance, but I didn't know whether to fall into Nepal or Tibet."

"Well, either way you'd be falling for the rest of your life, but Tibet is the greater distance so if you fell that way you'd live longer."

This conversation was starting to make sense—another reason not to stay at twenty-six thousand feet too long. The sun was already up and we wanted to get to Camp II today, five thousand feet lower. No longer using oxygen, we went over the top of the Geneva Spur and then down the other side, along the Yellow Band and onto the long traverse across the concave face of Lhotse which, because of our late start, was now focusing the sun's rays directly onto a team of tired climbers.

Camp III was an oasis—a place to rest, melt snow for drinks, and suck on a community oxygen tank left behind in one of the tents. Mook, looking very tired, was fully partaking of the delights when I arrived. I asked him if he was okay and he said no. Before I could follow up, Jim arrived. He asked him the same question but this time Mook said yes. I was the doctor and Jim was a climbing leader. Sometimes the answer to a question depends on who asks it.

The first rope length below Camp III was over slick hard ice. It was the pitch where Kami fell and I'm sure each climber was thinking about it on the descent. I couldn't help wondering where the exact spot was that Kami felt the horror of going over the edge.

Removing that thought, but not replacing it with any other, I rappelled mechanically down the ropes. At the end of one steep section, the slope angle lessened abruptly, becoming too gradual to continue the rappel. For a few seconds I was confused but then realized I was standing on the snow ramp. I was down.

In the morning I watched Camp II disappear. The expedition was coming off the mountain and the camp was being reduced to a series of overstuffed backpacks, most of them already on their way down to base camp on the backs of our team members. Only a few tents remained, just enough for those of us who were staying behind another day to finish packing up and cleaning up. How quickly our home reverted to what it really was—an insignificant flat spot on a barren moraine in a frozen wilderness.

According to their own radio reports, the part of our team that had already left was melting. They had gotten another late start, and the sun had been out for too long before they descended the icefall. Another radio call was coming up and I expected to hear Wally again, complaining good-naturedly about the heat. Todd was ready to suggest he go find some ice to suck on.

Instead we heard Lily's excited voice, followed by the tense but controlled voice of another climber. There was a lot of static and the message was breaking up. Each time we asked for it to be repeated, we were ignored. It was obvious our signal wasn't getting through at all. Finally we heard, "On the assumption that you can hear me, even though I can't hear you, I'll relate what's happening. Wally has fallen in a crevasse . . ."

Working from half sentences and unable to ask questions, we slowly put the story together, one agonizing bit at a time. Wally had been in the lead crossing a crevasse close to base camp. As he leaned on a guide rope for balance, the far anchor pulled out. The ice was soft and couldn't hold the screw. He lost his balance and toppled off the ladder, falling about sixty feet, landing upright but unconscious. Jim came up from behind, cut a length of rope from one of the fixed lines and, tying it to the middle of the ladder, lowered himself down into the crevasse.

Wally was wedged at the bottom but Jim was able to pass the rope through his harness. Wally regained consciousness and, with Jim pushing from below, he started up the crevasse by stepping into the ice on one side and pressing his back against the other wall for support. After a few feet though, the crevasse widened and, without the back wall to support him, Wally couldn't step up any higher.

Mook had continued on down to base camp to get help. Sherpas from the New Zealand expedition came back up with more rope and got to Jim and Wally while they were still stalled in the crevasse. Not bothering with any esoteric pulley principles, they dropped another line and hauled Wally to the surface.

Our injured climber was brought to base camp but the expedition doctor, me, was at Camp II, four thousand feet above him, trying to assess his condition over a staticky, intermittent radio. At least now the signal was working both ways so I could ask questions and give advice. Wally had two deep forehead lacerations and a swollen left arm that he didn't want to move. He was combative and confused. I had one of the climbers test Wally to see if he was also disoriented: When asked where he was, he replied, "New York." In answer to the climber's second question, "Do you know who I am?" Wally said, "Yeah, you're a loser."

"Well, one out of two isn't bad," I said dryly, but Wally needed evacuation.

I wanted to be on the helicopter with Wally but I was at Camp II, a Cwm and an icefall away. Descent to base camp now would be too dangerous. The sun had had all afternoon to soften the ice. To be safe I'd have to wait overnight for the icefall to refreeze, but the safest time for the helicopter to come would be early in the morning when the air was still and clear. To time it right, I would have to leave in the middle of the night—too soon and the ice wouldn't be hard enough, too late and I'd miss the flight.

Pete, Todd, Dawa, Nima Tashi, and I convened in the Sherpa kitchen tent (one of the few tents still up) to discuss the timing. Todd said the helicopter, if it came at all, would arrive about 7:00 A.M. Pete said the ice wouldn't be hard before 3:30 A.M. Dawa said, "Leave early because Dr. Ken very slow." Nima Tashi and I agreed with Dawa, but I couldn't leave until the ice was safe. We came to the conclusion that I'd have to fly as fast as the helicopter to make it down in time. When Nima Tashi volunteered to go with me, I said okay, as long as he promised not to slow me down.

Just before 2:00 A.M., in the cold and dark, Nima Tashi and I left the camp under a cloud-veiled half moon. The light reflecting off the ice was enough for Nima Tashi to move swiftly down the Cwm but even with my headlight switched on, I stumbled repeatedly, trying to maintain his pace.

There was no time for ego. I was traveling with an empty backpack, Nima Tashi carrying all of my gear plus his own. Down the Cwm we made good progress but I was moving in overdrive and tiring as we entered the icefall. The pace necessarily slowed as Nima Tashi went ahead to retap a screw or test a rope. Sometimes he would just look at the route, shake his head and take a detour. I wondered how you say "bad vibes" in Nepali.

We traveled through the coldest part of the night, past the worst of the overhanging seracs and stopped in a relatively open spot so I could catch my breath. To prevent overheating, I took off two layers of clothes and shamelessly handed them to Nima Tashi to carry for me. Still standing, we shared a frozen chocolate bar by smashing it against the ice to form edible-size pieces inside the wrapper, and then drank half a bottle of hot water each. Afraid we'd hear the helicopter at any moment, it was the ultimate eat and run.

It got light but we couldn't see. The moon disappeared but the fog that had veiled it remained. We knew we were close to base camp, at about the same altitude the helicopter pilot would need for a ceiling, so if we couldn't see the camp neither could he. That was good news because I was going to be late and now the helicopter will be too. Base camp radioed us that the pilot had come upvalley but had to divert to a nearby village because of the fog. The co-pilot said they were taking on more fuel and would wait for a hole in the clouds. I knew I would make it now. I was close enough that even if my teammates had to sit on the skids, they'd prevent the helicopter from taking off without me.

The noise of the rotors came just as we got down. A massive deafening machine suddenly disrupted the serene sky and overwhelmed us at base camp. For two months we hadn't seen anything like it or even heard any loud noise. The strange behemoth with its huge sweeping blades hovered a few feet above the ice. An alien jumped out to kick away a few rocks from the not-quite-flat-enough landing platform the Sherpas had built last night and finally the spaceship settled down, though the pilot kept the rotors spinning, afraid if he shut them off they wouldn't restart.

My tent had been cleaned out for me and my duffel bags already packed, but Lily had had the forethought to pull out a clean set of clothes, including underwear. In front of the helicopter, and in front of everybody, I changed out of my bulky climbing outfit as Sherpas led Wally past me and loaded him on board. In the swirling snowstorm created by the rotors, I said good-bye to the Sherpas and most of the climbers. I hugged Nima Tashi, not knowing if we'd ever see each other again. We yelled good-bye, though neither one of us could hear above the deafening noise.

The pilot had said he didn't want to be on the ground more than one minute and he was already down three. I boarded immediately after Wally and was surprised to see several climbers already inside with their luggage. It was a big helicopter and they were quick to seize an opportunity for an easy exit off the mountain.

The pilot and co-pilot were both on oxygen. Flying to this altitude without first acclimatizing and without supplemental oxygen would cause pulmonary edema in a few hours. If the helicopter stalled and couldn't be restarted, it would probably be fatal for them. Nevertheless, the co-pilot couldn't resist moving around the cabin shooting videos of the people from Everest. I wondered which of us were the aliens.

The door was snapped shut and the helicopter lifted off. I knelt down beside Wally, who was laid out alongside one wall. It was my first look at him. His face was puffy and his eye sockets were surrounded by rings of dried blood, giving him the look of a bloated raccoon. A bandage around his forehead covered two deep lacerations, there were splints taped to both arms, and an oxygen mask covered his face. He was alert but disoriented. I set about starting an intravenous line but had to stop when I saw the co-pilot open the door and throw out most of the luggage, including my duffel bags. Then, to my total confusion, the other climbers got up one by one, shook my hand, and jumped out of the helicopter. I hit my head against the porthole in my haste to look out, then saw that we were still hovering just a few feet off the ice. The pilot had taken on too much fuel while waiting to dash in for us and had to throw some flotsam overboard to get airborne again.

Less than two hours later, I was riding through hot brown air in the crowded streets of Kathmandu, bringing Wally to what must have been the world's oldest surviving X-ray machine. Wally didn't feel it was necessary—he wanted to stay at Camp II—but films showed that he had two skull fractures and two breaks in one of his forearm bones. The skull fractures were cracks that would heal on their own, but the forearm fragments were displaced with no contact between them. The arm would have to be set and casted. I brought Wally to a local clinic and did it myself. When I told Wally it came out well, he said he was "ready to go for the summit."

Going to the Yak & Yeti Hotel seemed like a better idea. I took a room with Wally so I could keep an eye on him, but it wasn't easy checking into the fanciest hotel in town without any identification. The desk clerk was polite but never quite believed my wild story about my passport and wallet being thrown out of a helicopter on Mount Everest.

I waited an hour and ten minutes for Wally to get out of the bath. When my turn came for the bathroom, I saw myself in the mirror for the first time in over two months. It was worse than I thought. My face was burned except for two white rings around the eyes where the goggles had covered them. My nose and cheeks were peeling in patches. I had a two-week growth of beard and my hair was projecting in all directions at once. The burn line ended at my neck and, except for my hands, the rest of my skin was pale. I had no chest, no butt, and spindly legs. I had lost thirty pounds and I looked like a scrawny chicken.

No sooner had I gotten into the warm water than the door banged open. Wally said, "I want to take a bath."

"Wally, you just took one."

"I don't care. I want to take one now!"

Wally was suffering from postconcussion syndrome. He would eventually return to his usual affable self but the injury and subsequent swelling of his brain were temporarily diminishing his higher cerebral functions. Memory, humor, and reasoning were impaired, as well as control over primitive instincts like aggression. I quickly stepped out of the tub and relinquished the bathroom to him again. There was no point in my taking a bath anyway, I reasoned, since I had nothing clean to change into. All my clothes were lost in the Khumbu.

Dinner at the hotel was served outside in the garden. I was especially sensitive to the warm night breeze and the delicate scent of the flowers. This morning I had awakened at Camp II and made a moonlit descent through the icefall. Breakfast there had been hot water and chocolate. After a wild helicopter ride, I set a fractured arm, then tucked my patient into bed. Now, with a dinner of poached salmon and Cabernet Sauvignon in a five-star hotel, I was finishing the longest day ever.

Exhilaration had prevented me from feeling tired. I began to think of the possibility of returning next year. The idea was exciting and that very excitement was disappointing. My goal had been to see if I could climb the world's tallest mountain. Coming within nine hundred feet and turning around only because of freak snow conditions, I now knew I could do it. It gave me the deep satisfaction and confidence I had anticipated it would. That should have been enough, but my eagerness to try again meant it wasn't.

Over the years, I've met many climbers derisively referred to as "peak-baggers," people who climb famous mountains just for the bragging rights. I always smugly reassured myself that I climbed for my own sense of accomplishment, not out of any desire to impress others. Would I go on a difficult or dangerous climb if I could never tell anyone about it? I firmly believed that I would, that it wouldn't matter if no one ever knew. But I was enthusiastic about returning for the last nine hundred feet of Everest because it did matter. Inner satisfaction was fine but I wanted the outer satisfaction too, the recognition that would only come if I summited. I was shallower than I thought. I wanted my trophy.

The dangers and the hardships of the mountain were already becoming blunted—a phenomenon all climbers experience, otherwise they'd never go back. This afternoon

I had seen Chantal in town. The pain in her ribs was completely gone and she was ready to climb again. She attributed the problem to wearing her bra too tight on summit day.

Chantal still looked pretty good, although not as good as she looked on the mountain. Everything seems to look better on the mountain, but it's a scene painted in acrylics and after a while I long to see the more subtle but richer blend of colors that paint real life.

The expedition wasn't quite over yet. The transition would come in a few minutes when I called Josiane. It was getting late enough on this side of the world that it wouldn't be too early on the other. I wouldn't see the colors yet but I'd hear the music. Connecting the phone would be like dropping a needle onto an already-spinning record. The music would be in midsong, complete with melody and full harmonics. When I heard the familiar tune, I'd begin to be home.

"Kenny! You just got me. I was on my way out the door to take the kids to school."

She surprised me by saying she was proud of me for having the courage to turn around so close to the top—even prouder than if I had summited. It confirmed her feeling that I could control the risk and allayed her fear that I didn't recognize all I had at home. She said "For us, you summited. The last nine hundred feet don't make any difference."

Josiane always knew what to say. I lay back in bed on a folded-up white yak-wool sweater that I had gotten in town today. I had seen it in a shop window and recognized it immediately as the one Josiane was wearing in my oxygen-enriched dream at Camp III. Resting my head on the soft sweater, I imagined Josiane was inside.

She was right. I didn't need another nine hundred feet of ice to make my life complete. In my head and in my heart, I agreed. Finally letting the fatigue of the day and of the expedition overwhelm me, I drifted off into sleep, but I could feel the countercurrent that would be drawing me back to Everest yet again.

CHAPTER
11

In ancient times people believed a comet was the harbinger of disaster. It seemed like nonsense as my family and I searched the sky over New York for Hyakutake. When we found it, it set our faces aglow with excitement. The comet was a once-in-a-lifetime cosmic show.

That was two weeks earlier, and since then I'd returned to the other side of the planet. The comet was still overhead. Here at base camp, on this remote mountain unchanged for thousands of years, the streaming tail of white light dominated the sky. The comet had an ominous power and presence that made me wonder if the ancients who saw it this way understood it better than we did.

Hyakutake added to my doubts about being here. The many reasons to stay at home had to be fended off by an unshakable sense of purpose. It's never easy to get away. This year, with uncertain motivation, my pieces didn't fall into place easily, as though I had forced something not meant to happen. I had already proven to myself I could climb Everest. This time I was here merely to summit—a far less worthy undertaking for which Everest might not have the patience to indulge me. I was afraid of wearing out my welcome, and seeing a comet over this mountain gave cosmic magnitude to my personal misgivings.

Earthlings are not powerless, however, to affect their fate. Instead of taking the low road through Nima Tashi's village of Pangboché as we usually did on our approach march, this year our expedition was directed up a hill to a neat square stone house crowned with a copper roof. Nima Tashi asked us to wait outside while he went off to get the village lama, who was out blessing crops. A few minutes later an old man in red and orange robes put a heavy iron key in a heavy wooden door and opened the monastery.

Inside, it was dark except for a small skylight which illuminated wooden walls completely covered with brightly colored paintings of Buddha and all the Tibetan gods. We took seats on low carpet-covered benches and listened as the lama chanted and beat a yak-skin drum suspended from the ceiling. A rope was ingeniously attached to the drum stick so that it closed and opened a cymbal with each stroke. The lama was a one-man band.

Nima Tashi had arranged this puja in my honor—a special prayer ceremony to show his gratitude to me and to protect our expedition. The incessant drum and cymbal beat dominated the small dark room, creating a hypnotic effect. Nima Tashi stepped to the center to say a prayer, then lit a candle and hung his prayer shawl around a black wooden tiger head with red eyes that glowed in the dark. He motioned for me to hang my shawl there as well, and then for the others to follow. When we finished, the music stopped suddenly and the spell was broken. The puja had gone well. Nima Tashi relaxed and served each of us hot tea from a bottle. The lama would say a prayer and keep a candle burning for us every day of the expedition.

Other spirits also needed to be reckoned with. At the top of a steep slope along a bleak, desolate ridgeline was the Sherpa memorial. In previous years we'd passed by the row of stone monuments because it was always too windy to stop. This year we stopped anyway. Each time a Sherpa dies in the mountains a new monument is erected. The last one along the line was Kami's, and I draped a prayer shawl around it.

Hyakutake wasn't the only visitor to Everest this year, though admittedly it came the farthest distance to get here. Our camp was the closest to the comet, then right below us, as usual, was Rob Hall's New Zealand team. Close below them was another American team led by Scott Fischer, and an IMAX film team led by Dave Breashears, here to film a scripted and rehearsed movie with Everest playing a supporting role.

Our expedition was much smaller than the others. Besides our Sherpas, there was Todd, Pete, Jim, and me and two newcomers: Steve Bridges, an electronics engineer from Arizona, and Charles Corfield, an English mathematician living in San Francisco who made Silicon Valley investments. Todd and Pete and some of the Sherpas had been here for weeks already, staking a claim on the ice and carving out a camp. The rest of us came in today, taking twelve days to get here instead of the usual ten. Heavy snows had slowed yak traffic, forcing our leisurely pace. We couldn't arrive ahead of the yak train since it was carrying the supplies we'd need to stay on the mountain. Nevertheless, we left the yaks behind at Gorak Shep this morning to be sure we got to camp early. Sherpas had radioed us yesterday that today at 11:00 A.M. would be the most auspicious time for the official expedition puja. The yaks could show up later; we didn't want to miss a blessing.

We were making our way through the lower base camps when the ceremonies started, each team lighting juniper at its own lhapso at precisely eleven o'clock. I waved hello as I passed Frank, who was sitting with the New Zealand team, and then continued on to my puja, going nonstop from Gorak Shep to a rock in front of the lhapso. Frank had gone with the New Zealanders this year, hoping to change his luck. When I went down to visit him, the expedition was taking a group photo and Frank was gone. He had said he had to go to the bathroom, but Frank was superstitious about avoiding team photos. He had seen too many where one or another person was pointed to as not having made it back. Immediately after the photo he returned, not expecting the group to be taking a second one. I forced him to stay this time and he reluctantly became part of the official record. He said, "The only shot I wanted to be in was the summit photo."

"You should have come with us then, Frank."

"No, I'll be more comfortable with a British-style group."

"I don't know about that. We have no group photo and we even have a British guy with us. You wouldn't be the only one who talks funny."

Easily I lapsed into the familiar routine of base camp: setting up the medical tent and taking care of the myriad illnesses and injuries while at the same time trying to breathe, eat, and stay warm. By now, I knew most of the Sherpas and even recognized some of the yaks from last year. There were, however, new rules to get used to, one of which required some amount of toilet training. The Nepalese government, in their infinite wisdom, decreed that our solid waste had to be taken off the mountain. That meant that we couldn't just use a crevasse or dig a deep hole. The hole had to be shaped so that a barrel could be fitted inside. Only the climbers' waste, however, had to be in barrels. The Sherpas' waste didn't count. They could (and did) go anywhere they wanted. They were considered part of the natural environment and we were not. Never mind that they wouldn't be here either if it wasn't for us.

When the barrel was filled, it had to be removed, replaced, and then transported for disposal all the way to Kathmandu—where it would no doubt be dumped in the street like all the other waste there. This was considered more environmentally sound than leaving it frozen in the ice in an uninhabited region.

To keep transport volume and weight down, only solid waste, not liquid had to be collected. This was succinctly explained on a sign outside the outhouse that said "Don't Pee in the Barrel."

As usual, the food was better at the New Zealand camp, so I mooched a meal there whenever I could. This was the first time Jan wasn't around and I missed my medical associate. Jan and Rob were married now and Rob said she was home waiting for their first baby. Rob told me, "Jan said, 'When you see Ken tell him hello and then make sure he gets to the summit this time—even if you have to kick his ass up there.'"

I was sure Jan didn't put it exactly that way but I appreciated the thought. Usually right after Everest Rob goes off and tries another mountain, but this year he'd be flying straight home. The baby was due in three months and Rob said, "I promised Jan I'll arrive before the baby does."

Doug Hansen, the postman from Seattle, was back again. I had treated him at Camp II last year for frostbitten toes but it was a mild case and he said they had fully recovered. Mike Groom, one of Rob's guides, said he never worried about his toes anymore—he lost them all to frostbite years ago.

Andy Harris was Rob's other guide and this was his first trip to the Himalayas. It was also the first time here for a friendly Texan named Beck Weathers, a pathologist with a lot of climbing experience elsewhere. Stuart Hutchison was a doctor too—a cardiologist. I had met him on the trail when he was stopped for two days by diarrhea. And there was Yasuko Namba, a Japanese woman, very shy and unassuming though she had already climbed the highest peaks on the other six continents.

The consensus was that the icefall was a little easier than last year, and a few days later I was finding out for myself on my first run. It did seem less jumbled and more wavy than last time, as if the Cwm had rolled down lower into the falls. After a tough five hours, I had to agree with the consensus although, sitting outside Camp I trying to catch my breath, I would have used the term *less hard* rather than *easier*.

Rhythm of movement on a big mountain is driven by weather and terrain, leading expeditions to the same place at the same time. The snow wall, on which I was sitting while it was still being completed by my less-tired teammates, was a front-row seat for the ice show going on right below me. The IMAX movie team was setting up camp, returning after a day of shooting prerehearsed action scenes in the icefall. Besides the Sherpas with the usual climbing equipment, there was one carrying a huge folded metal tripod and another with a heavy metal box containing the enormous camera. After them came two nice-looking female climbers, the film's starlets. Araceli Segarra was from Spain, a blonde with a big smile. Sumiyo Tsuzuki was Japanese—tall, thin, and reserved. Though the camps were very close and we were certainly trying, it was hard to get a good look at the discreet Sumiyo. Araceli, on the other hand, was a natural performer. She was aware of her audience and made a big show out of walking up to our camp to borrow a shovel. She introduced herself to everyone, put the shovel over her shoulder, and then walked back self-consciously, knowing we were all watching her.

Later, the director, Dave Breashears, came by. A cinematographer who had summited Everest twice and was well known in climbing circles, Dave was already friendly with Todd and Pete, so he sat down on the ice to socialize.

Todd, being a bachelor, immediately asked Dave, "How did you pick the girls?"

The answer was interesting. He wanted a Spanish climber because this year there was going to be an international IMAX film festival in Barcelona. He wanted a Japanese climber because there were more IMAX theaters in Japan than anywhere else.

"What about their climbing ability?"

"We thought about that."

"What about their looks?"

"No, that didn't hurt their chances any."

Before leaving, Dave said he wanted to keep our shovel a little longer to dig a latrine for his group.

Todd said, "So that's what a famous international film director does."

Early light was the best illumination for the top of the icefall, so in the morning at breakfast we leaned back against our snow wall and watched the IMAX team shoot a scene. The two women were on the set along with the two male stars, Ed Viesturs, an American superclimber, and Jamling, the son of Tenzing Norgay, the Sherpa who summited Everest with Edmund Hillary. They put on huge backpacks, puffed out by foam pads inside and worn so that the brand name was clearly visible since the company was paying extra for it. The camera was set up as they walked down over the sloping edge of the icefall, just out of sight. When Dave yelled "Action!" the four climbers appeared out of the ice-fall, each wearing a different colored jacket for easy identifi-cation. They moved with slow plodding steps, bent forward from the weight of their packs and tired after having just climbed from base camp. They didn't have to endure very long though, since a magazine of film lasts only ninety sec-onds. Soon Dave yelled, "Cut! Thank you." With that, all four climbers suddenly straightened up and strode quickly back to camp.

I asked Todd what we would do for entertainment now, but I didn't have to worry. Just then Charles came out of his tent wearing white long underwear and climbing boots. Heading down the hill in a hurry, he was carrying a roll of toilet paper with the end streaming along behind him. It was the "phantom of the latrine"—too bad Dave didn't have his camera reloaded yet. The lower half of Charles disap-peared on the other side of a small snow wall where there was a big garbage bag for us to use. Even above the icefall we were supposed to carry out our solid waste. We complied, more or less, but we all wanted to know who the inspector was who was going to come up here to check, and how he was going to identify the miscreants. Anyway, Dave's latrine was a good effort and, before moving up the Cwm, we con-gratulated the movie director on his heretofore unknown talent, still not fully appreciated by Hollywood.

Camp II greeted us with a stiff wind. Our host was Dawa, who had actually moved in here, living at 21,000 feet for the duration of the expedition so that he could maintain the camp by digging out the tent whenever snow arrived and by preparing meals whenever Sherpas or climbers arrived. He was better at digging. In the middle of lunch, which no one was eating anyway, the wind started blowing the tent around. One of the outside support poles came apart and the roof sagged in on our heads. Todd tried to fix it from the inside while Jim ran out to work on it from the outside. The tent wall was like a filled sail that the wind was lifting off the ground but they were managing to hold it down. Todd yelled for the rest of us to go out and check the other tents. The clear sunny day had suddenly turned opaque and a piercing cold wind was whipping snow sideways into our faces. We could hardly see the tents, but none seemed ready to take off, though they were flapping wildly. To keep them on the ground, we rolled large stones inside and then got in ourselves, leaving our boots on so we could get out in a hurry if the tent started tumbling. I kept my knife in my hand in case the walls collapsed and I had to cut myself out.

During a brief lull in the wind we looked out to survey the damage. Our camp was intact. We looked over to the New Zealand camp and saw their blue tents were valiantly being held down by two Sherpas, the rest of the expedition having moved up to Camp III today. Their camp seemed intact too, until we noticed one tent missing and a large blue balloon wafting above the moraine.

All night long the wind prevented us from sleeping, beating the tents with a constant flapping noise. Charles and I were in one tent; Steve was in another by himself, except for some extra rocks. I had put him in "isolation" because of a persistent productive cough. In the morning the tent was still flapping and Steve was still coughing. I was so tired I thought I hadn't slept at all until I remembered being awakened by Charles, who shined his headlight in my face to tell me he had diarrhea.

After adding more rope and more ballast to the tents, we finished—or chose not to finish—a breakfast of cold cereal in water. We left Todd, Dawa, and a skeleton crew to guard the tents while the team headed up to Camp III to drop supplies and acclimatize on a one-night stand. This was my first trip up the Lhotse Face this season and again it looked awesome and foreboding. I had to remind myself that I'd done this several times before, in order to not be intimidated by it.

The huge permanent crevasse at the base of Lhotse was partially filled by heavy snowfall this season. There was no trace, except a mental one, of where Kami's body had come to rest. We were able to cross the crevasse by jumaring up a steep ice bridge which directly connected the lower edge of the crevasse to the top of the snow ramp, avoiding the usual long detour. It made the route shorter but added a long vertical section right at the beginning, leaving us tired by the time we reached the start of the face. The slope fell back to its usual relentless angle, but just gradual enough to hold a thin accumulation of snow on top of the ice. It made the footing a little easier but it didn't make Lhotse any smaller.

Above us we could see a thundering herd on the ropes. The New Zealand team was on its way down from III. We'd have to pass each other—not an easy thing to do when you're all standing at a 45-degree angle connected to the slope by a single continuous line. The safest way is for the person moving up to stop at an anchoring screw while the person coming down reaches around and hooks in below him, hopefully without detaching from the same anchor until he's securely clipped in again.

It's a moment that requires close contact and brings you face-to-face with every climber going in the other direction. As one bearded climber was preparing to pass me, I heard Frank call down from above. "Jon, that's the doctor I was telling you about."

I realized that this guy must be Jon Krakauer, the writer with the New Zealand expedition. Frank had been trying to interest him in doing a story about Nima Tashi and me and was anxious for us to meet. Despite the absurd circumstances, Jon had the gentility to take his glove off to shake my hand. We said we'd talk more about it later, but before we were both off the mountain Jon would have a much bigger story to write about.

The Taiwanese team, none of whose members I knew, was also descending from Camp III. One by one I passed the unfamiliar faces until one member stopped alongside me and said, "Here, Dr. Sab, have some water." I didn't know him but he knew me, and I accepted his thoughtful offer.

I hadn't thought it possible but Camp III looked worse than last year—narrower, more precarious, and slanting to one side. Pete tried to level it by chopping away with his ax, sending chunks of ice skittering down the slope. A few minutes later a climber came up the rope like a disgruntled neighbor. His camp was below ours and one of his team members had already been hit in the arm. He told Pete to stop the bombardment.

After our overnight stay for acclimatization, I redescended to the luxury of Camp II. I was looking forward to recuperating in my flat-bottomed tent when Todd came out to greet me. He said, "A Sherpa up here on Scott Fischer's team might have pulmonary edema. Their doctor's at base trying to control the situation but I think they need some help."

That wasn't the greeting I had expected. My beeper had gone off.

I didn't even go to my tent. I just dropped my gear on the rocks and started up the moraine to their camp, along with Pete and Jim. We found Ngawang in their cook tent sitting upright on a mat on the floor. He was unable to lie down, and he had a rapid pulse and a blue color. He was on oxygen and breathing deeply. Jim noticed right away that the tank wasn't connected properly, and when he fixed it, the blue color disappeared. I could hear the noise in Ngawang's lungs just by putting my ear to his chest.

"This guy has got flagrant pulmonary edema," I radioed to Ingrid Hunt, their base camp doctor.

She said, "He's already been given nifedipine, dexamethasone, and diamox, plus two sessions in a Gamoff bag; he should be improving."

"Take my word for it," I assured her, "he looks terrible."

Ingrid wasn't sure he needed to be brought down but she wasn't examining him. I was, and he did. As we would say at home, you can't defer responsibility to another doctor over the phone (or radio), so I had to be in charge. Only three of Scott's climbers and a few Sherpas were at the camp. Scott and his two guides were at base with the rest of the team. There would be just enough manpower to get Ngawang down but far short of enough time to do it before nightfall. Too many hours had been lost already.

As the rescuers were leaving, Jim got on the radio to coordinate a second team that would start up from base to take the relay. With only about three hours until sunset, the icefall descent would be in the dark—difficult and dangerous. There was enough daylight to make it to Camp I but that was only two thousand feet lower. An overnight stop there would probably mean there would be no need for a rescue in the morning. To save Ngawang I felt they had to get all the way to base camp, but it wasn't me who would be taking the risk.

I drew up some medications and wrote out a list of instructions on how and when to give them. The rescuers started off on their long hard journey, and Jim and I went back to our camp. Tomorrow we'd be descending to base ourselves; we'll have to wait until then to find out what happened.

In the morning, as I was nearing the bottom of the icefall, I passed Scott on his way up. He thanked me for taking charge of the situation yesterday. Ngawang was still alive and everyone had made it down safely. I was relieved to hear it, but suprised that the team leader was going up the icefall when he had a sick Sherpa below.

After settling in at base camp, I took a walk with Pete to Scott's camp to find out what was going on. Lopsang, who had worked with Rob last year and was back this year as Scott's head Sherpa, served us hot tea and led us to a tent in a corner of the camp. Inside we found Ngawang lying by himself on a mattress. Pete and I were shocked. Although he sounded drier than yesterday, one lung had developed a small dead spot where no air was moving. It probably meant he was getting pneumonia.

Lopsang went to get Ingrid and we all sat down together along with Neal Beidleman, Scott's guide who had taken the re-lay and led the rescue through the icefall. Ngawang needed oxygen, antibiotics, and evacuation. Ingrid seemed over-whelmed—it was her first time at base camp—so Pete volun-teered to have us take care of him in our camp. Though I was very willing to help out and would have taken over if I thought it was necessary, it seemed they could handle it themselves with some advice. Besides, I wasn't eager for another major distrac-tion, especially from a different expedition. Pete sensed my lack of enthusiasm and didn't repeat the offer a second time.

The air between first light and sunrise was still and cold. Base camp was quiet and it was a peaceful time to walk around. Depending on the weather, we'd be here for about five days to rest, and prepare for the summit attempt. Checking my medical tent early one morning I found some-one sleeping inside. His clothes were disheveled and his head was wrapped in rags. As we got closer to summit day, a lot of strange people were being drawn to the camps.

Especially porters. Usually once they dropped their supplies they took their yaks and left, but for days now they were all hanging around trying to make "big shit money." The government was paying eight hundred rupees (fourteen dollars) for every full barrel brought down the mountain to Namché to be flown out by helicopter. Each time an outhouse was emptied, there was fierce competition to be a "shit-carry man." The porters were attracted to the stuff like flies.

In the mess tent at mealtime I learned that the vagrant in the medical tent was a college graduate student—a Nepali surveyor who had come up to help monitor our latest GPS equipment if and when we ever get it up on top. He may have regretted joining us for lunch, though. It was a pot of macaroni which could be served only by cutting it into blocks. Charles tossed a piece out the door to see if one of the scavenging ravens could swallow it. Instead of reporting back that the bird didn't eat it, he said, "Apparently it's not within the scope of its forage pattern."

I said, "Charles, you're a nerd. How can someone like you climb faster than me?"

A more serious question was what to do with Scott's Sherpa. A few days of windy and cloudy skies meant Ngawang couldn't be flown out so he was carried down to the HRA clinic in Pheriché. The doctors there reported back that he wasn't doing well and had to be intubated (a tube inserted in his throat) to help him breathe. Later we heard he was flown out to Kathmandu.

The sun came out very early one day but it was just a trick. By the time I got out to wash, the sun was gone and before I got back to my tent, it was snowing. The sudden drop in barometric pressure was too much for a vacuum-packed container of raisins, which exploded in my tent. It seemed like a good day to stay inside until Ong-Chu came to tell me that Todd, who was at Camp II, wanted to speak to me on the radio. I stopped picking raisins off the ceiling and went out to take the call.

Nima Tashi, while trying to make a carry to Camp IV, had turned around because of pain in his ankle. He was back at Camp II now and Todd needed advice. The ankle was brittle, and if it had absorbed too much stress it may have broken. Sherpas don't turn around without good reason.

I told Todd how to apply a bandage so that it would reduce the swelling and give maximum support, then waited on standby while he did it. He came back on a few minutes later to say, "It looks better than if you wrapped it."

"We'll see about that when he gets down here." We laughed, but a serious injury to Nima Tashi would be a serious blow to our expedition, and to me personally. His recovery was one of my proudest accomplishments, he was my guardian angel, and he was my friend.

The next morning we were dining al fresco. The sun had finally shown up and we took advantage of it by having breakfast on the rocks. The warm air even emboldened me to shave. After a painful hour of pulling hairs and unclogging the razor with my knife after each stroke, the final result was pretty good. It wasn't vanity that made me shave. Too much hair on my face might loosen the seal on my oxygen mask. I was getting ready for summit day.

Just as I finished, Nima Tashi appeared out of the icefall. He had completely ignored my advice to rest a day before descending and said that he felt much better since the bandage was on. I took him into the medical tent for an examination while everyone waited outside. A few minutes later I emerged with the verdict. "Well, Todd, I've got to admit you did a good job wrapping the fused ankle . . ."

Todd smiled proudly.

". . . but next time maybe you want to wrap the one he injured."

The smile collapsed into confusion until I explained. Todd and I and everyone else had assumed the problem was with the fused ankle, but Nima Tashi's pain was in the other ankle. He thought it was strange that Todd wrapped the "wrong" ankle yesterday but didn't say anything because he assumed that Todd and Dr. Ken knew what they were doing. Today he felt reassured that we were right since his ankle felt much better.

Sherpas are so tough and so anxious not to look weak that you have to be very careful in believing their stories, but my exam had confirmed what he said. There was some residual swelling over the "good" ankle and no sign of damage to the fused one. He had had an overuse injury, his good leg compensating for the bad one as he carried a heavy load up Lhotse. The bandage may have actually helped by allowing him to bear more weight on the fused side. A few days' rest and he should be ready for a summit bid. Everyone was relieved, especially me.

On to the next problem: the rotten, painful tooth of Ang Dorje, the lead climbing Sherpa of the New Zealand team. They were leaving on their summit bid tomorrow and Rob asked if I could help. I had a great set of new dental instruments and this would be the perfect opportunity to try them out, especially since I wanted to come by anyway to wish them all luck. This was exciting. I had never been a dentist before.

Waiting for Ang Dorje to arrive, I shared tea and crackers with Rob and most of the members of the team as they came in and out. There was tension in the air. Most of the climbers were subdued; some covered their nervousness with little jokes. Rob had the usual twinkle in his eyes and was the only one who looked fully at ease. Mountains were his natural element.

By the fifth cup of tea, it had become obvious that Ang Dorje wasn't going to show. After the eighth, another Sherpa came in to tell us that Ang Dorje said his tooth wasn't hurting anymore. Our patient had chickened out, but at least I had gotten the chance to visit with the New Zealanders—some of them, it would turn out, for the last time.

By sunrise the New Zealand team was gone, as was Scott Fischer's team except for a few stragglers. Our team would be leaving tomorrow. There was quiet activity around the camp as each of us laid out clothes and equipment, making sure everything worked. Jim noticed a tear in my climbing boot and took it to his tent to glue and tape. Todd gave me an extra lithium bulb for my headlight. I put on fresh underwear and socks and arranged my pack, trying to figure out a way to make its total weight less than what I was putting inside. Jim returned, satisfied with his repair of my boot but curious as to how raisins had gotten in there.

My medical supplies were long-since neatly arranged, but at the last minute people were requesting pills and items to carry personally so I made a trip to the medical tent to put together individual packets. While I was there a climber brought in Mingma, a climbing Sherpa who had fallen yesterday into a small crevasse. Today his back was hurting. I thought he might have bruised his kidneys but it didn't seem serious. I told him the next time he peed he should bring me some in a cup. He thought that was the funniest thing he had ever heard and that made us all laugh.

Mingma left but the climber hung around while I resumed making up packets. Although he was a very experienced climber, I sensed he wanted to talk to me so I took a break. He said he was developing a case of shingles brought on by stress—not from climbing but from his marriage. He was going through a tough time and even here on the mountain he wasn't mentally away from it.

Mingma interrupted us, coming into the tent with a big smile and a cup of pee in his hands. There was no blood in it so I reassured him he was okay.

The climber and I resumed our conversation. I told him it would be better if the mountain was more scary to him, as it was to me. Mental stresses from a mountain are basic and even healthy, unlike the complex stresses from a marriage. If you're preoccupied with survival, there is no room for other thoughts.

The morning of our ascent began at 3:45 with the familiar clang of a spoon against an oxygen cylinder. I read my "secret notes" although I knew them all by heart already, then tucked them into my inside pocket along with the family dolls. My personal ritual completed, I went out to the lhapso to perform the team ritual of inhaling juniper smoke and throwing rice on the fire.

There was no wind and the air was just cold enough to keep the ice solidly frozen—perfect conditions for climbing. Pete led the way and did the incidental road work, as he called it, testing ropes and hammering in questionable anchors. Each successive section marked out in my mind came sooner than expected. I was making good progress. Camp I appeared not long after sunrise.

Lying on our packs outside the tents, we took in the sun and the vast spectacular view from the top of the icefall. The stillness was broken occasionally by a dot of motion which progressed to a figure and then to a person we could recognize as she or he came up alongside.

Sandy Pittman paused for a few minutes of friendly conversation to break the boredom of the climb before continuing on into the Cwm. She was with Scott's team this year but Sandy and I met three years ago when we were on the same Everest expedition. She was a climber most of her life but she became a prominent New York socialite after her husband founded MTV. Sandy was rich and well-connected, and quick to let you know it. That annoying habit obscured her impressive climbing credentials, and when disaster struck the Fischer team, she became an easy target.

The next climber to come by looked like Rudolph Nureyev but it was Scott's Russian guide, Anatoli Boukreev. He seemed to dance over the ice and as he reached us we marvelled that he had come through the icefall wearing sneakers.

Scott himself passed by a few minutes later acting as sweeper. The group was moving directly up to Camp II today to unite with the rest of the team. Scott had some discouraging news from Kathmandu. Ngawang was very close to death.

Doctors always have a reflex reaction when one of their patients dies: Should I have done something different? My first year here I might have had gnawing self-doubt but by now I had more confidence—enough to be able to think of poor Ngawang rather than myself.

It didn't take long until fog came up the valley, taking away the sun and ruining our view. My sleeping bag had been draped over the top of my tent to serve as insulation from the hot sun but quickly I had to pull it inside so it wouldn't fill with the snow that suddenly started falling.

One day and many crevasses later we arrived at Camp II. Although the same place as before, it was now the launching pad for the summit push—the last station where we could rest and make minor adjustments while watching the weather to time our liftoff. The forecast had looked promising from here this morning so Rob's team and Scott's team, as well as two Taiwanese climbers, moved up to III today. The IMAX team was already at III, but from their vantage point it looked too windy to go higher up. They decided instead to come back down here to wait things out. The consensus among our Sherpas was also too much wind. If they didn't like the weather, then we didn't like the weather so we put the countdown on hold by making the next day a rest day.

Sitting in camp with nobody sick and not much to do, I was checking for the third time that my oxygen mask fit snugly and the regulator worked smoothly when I heard that, in fact, there was somebody sick, but he wasn't here at Camp II. Sherpas from the IMAX team radioed Dave that they were descending Lhotse with Chen Yu Nan, an injured Taiwanese they had found at Camp III. This morning he had left his tent early to go to the bathroom without putting on his crampons. He slipped and fell into a crevasse. He lay there awhile before being discovered, but after he was pulled out he seemed to be okay. Makalu Gau, the team leader and the only other Taiwanese up there, elected to continue the climb alone, though that meant leaving Yu Nan alone too.

When the Sherpas came upon him, his condition had deteriorated but he was still able to walk. They hooked him into the ropes and, with some difficulty, were helping him descend. There were no other details yet but three possibilities came to mind immediately: this could be a subdural hematoma, this could be a ruptured spleen, this could end my chance for the summit.

I concentrated on the first two possibilities. I had no IV fluids and few injectibles—they freeze too easily at this altitude. I would have to make the most out of pills and bandages. The third possibility would take care of itself one way or the other.

The next radio report was that the Sherpas were coming down alone: Yu Nan had collapsed and died. The Sherpas were unwilling to touch him, fearing it would be bad karma. Confirmation of the report was sickeningly obvious, as a body could be seen against the Lhotse Face dangling from the ropes.

Dave and Ed climbed up to end the spectacle. They wrapped the body in a sleeping bag, lowered it down the fixed lines, and left it on the ice just outside camp. Yu Nan needed an undertaker, not a doctor. I was back to being a climber again.

A hailstorm blew through camp, ending the afternoon. Higher up, though, the wind had apparently quieted down and both Rob and Scott were able to move their teams up to the Col. They were resting at Camp IV along with Makalu, who was undeterred despite the death of his climbing partner. When advised of Yu Nan's death, his only response was "Okay, thank you." At about midnight, if the weather looked good, they'd all be going for the summit. Here at II, the IMAX team would be taking another day to regroup but our team was ready, so if our Sherpa weathermen approved, we'd try to move up to III in the morning. Summiting Everest had now come down to needing three good days in a row plus some luck.

CHAPTER

12

By sunrise we were en route. Though it was cold and windy when I left Camp II, I had intentionally under-dressed, knowing that I move a lot faster when I'm a little bit cold. I expected the air to warm after the sun came up, but as I approached the vertical section bridging the crevasse I was just too cold and had to add a layer before starting up. I climbed strongly, by my standards. This part of the route was becoming familiar territory and I didn't waste much energy on anxiety or uncertainty, though not retaining any fear would have required losing touch with reality.

Todd was the first to reach Camp III. By the time I got there he was busy trying to undercut the narrow platform so the tent would lie flat. I was too tired to help and with no place to stand, I clipped in to the other end of the tent and sat against the edge with my feet hanging over the two-thousand-foot drop. Steve came up and sat alongside me but didn't clip in right away so I did it for him.

"I'm okay like this," he said as I was reaching over.

"Yeah," I answered, "that was probably what Yu Nan said too."

Though crumpled together in a two-man tent, the three of us were having a tough time staying warm. The wind never relaxed and the sun only rarely found its way through the clouds. Heat and light would fill the tent momentarily, only to be repeatedly blown out by the wind.

Todd hung a stove inside the tent entrance, out of the wind, and boiled snow to heat the frozen food packets. Fuel was in short supply so cooking times had to be shortened, a recipe modification I became aware of as I swallowed the ice balls of my partially thawed meal. Lying on one elbow inside my sleeping bag as I ate, I waited for our scheduled radio call to hear the news of the summit attempt going on two thousand feet above us.

It wasn't what we wanted to hear. Rob, his two guides Mike and Andy, and three others had reached the top. There was jubilation and champagne at base camp far below. But five of the group, including Frank and Beck, had turned back early and the others hadn't summited until two-thirty—an hour and a half later than Rob's own cutoff rule. Conditions must be tough up there, I thought, and there wasn't much daylight left. I recalled uneasily that I had treated most of the New Zealand team after their summit attempt last year when they had stayed out too late.

Clouds moved in low over our heads, blocking our view of the South Col. We left the radio on standby, hoping to hear soon that everyone was back safely. Instead there was a long silence as it slowly got dark outside. When the radio did crackle on again, we heard a chilling report: Rob had waited overlong to descend with Doug Hansen, the last one up. Doug was now out of oxygen and too exhausted to descend the Hillary Step, a moderately difficult rock face just below the summit. The rest of the New Zealand team was also having trouble getting back. Scott Fischer's team, with the curious exception of Scott, had all summited but none of them had been heard from since. Nor was there any word on the Taiwanese, Makalu. Climbers were still strung out all over the mountain and apparently some hadn't yet descended much below the summit. They would all soon be exhausted and out of oxygen, if they weren't already. Those of us at Camp III could hardly stand the cold and wind, and we were in sleeping bags and tents. The night passed with us in fitful sleep, unable or unwilling to think about what was happening to the exposed climbers several thousand feet above us.

The radio came on at 5:00 A.M. and we awoke to the horror story we didn't want to imagine. Rob had been out all night with Doug, who was now too weak to move. Rob was also long since out of oxygen and could hardly move himself. He didn't say where they were, but climbers had seen a headlight just above the Hillary Step. They had made no progress overnight.

The entire Scott Fischer team had still not been heard from, nor had anyone heard from Makalu. On the New Zealand team, Jon Krakauer had summited and gotten back to his tent. He had a radio but didn't much know what was going on except that it was very cold and there was a whiteout with high winds and blowing snow. He couldn't see outside his tent. That meant that the people who were trying to make it back after having been out all night wouldn't be able to find the camp.

Jon said Andy had been right behind him and also had a radio but as of yet no one had heard from him. Mike, the other guide, was back at IV but was hypothermic and frostbitten. Jon hadn't seen Yasuko since shortly after they all summited, but he had passed Beck on the way down. Beck hadn't summited but he hadn't returned either. There was no word on Frank, and I remembered that day in base camp when he had tried to avoid the team photo but had gotten

caught in it anyway. I had laughed then about his super-
stition.

More radio reports came in—most of them conflicting,
all of them confusing. Apparently, though, there were about
eighteen people who still hadn't returned to Camp IV. The
temperature had plummeted overnight and the wind was
blowing snow into our tents right through the fabric. So
loud was the noise and so violent the flapping of our two
tents that it was impossible to talk between them even by
shouting. We had to use our radios to communicate and
formulate a rescue plan.

Despite the wind, Todd in our tent and Pete in the other
simultaneously prepared to make their way up to the South
Col. They skipped any discussion of whether they should
go, beginning their radio contact with questions of how
quickly they could get started and what they should bring.
As Todd got ready, I gave him the few medications we had,
our extra pairs of gloves, and some quick advice on treating
the medical conditions he and Pete would be likely to encounter among the survivors. Having worked together with
them for years, I was confident they could take good care of
anyone they found alive but reminded them to be extremely
careful before deciding that someone wasn't.

Just before setting off, they directed their radios down
the mountain speaking first to Dave at Camp II and then to
base camp. Dave explained where he had stashed oxygen,
fuel, and fresh radio batteries on the Col and then told them
to take whatever they needed. To base camp they read off a
list of medical supplies I had prepared, which I wanted
brought up to Camp II as soon as possible. Then they asked,
if possible, for a message to be passed up to Rob. I expected
something to the effect of "Help is on the way," but instead
what I heard was, "Tell Rob that the situation is hopeless for
both of them if they stay together. He should abandon Doug

and try to get himself down. Better to save one than lose two."

In a swirl of wind and cold, Todd crawled out the tent door and we watched as he and Pete started up the ropes. The air was clear where we were, but the clouds that had rolled in yesterday were still above our heads. Surface snow, stirred up by the wind, mixed with the clouds to form a whiteout completely obscuring the South Col. Todd and Pete climbed up steadily and disappeared into the maelstrom.

We zipped shut the tent door. In the relative calm inside, Jim radioed our Sherpas at Camp II, and asked them to try to come up to the Col to help. The Sherpas refused, saying it was too dangerous to be on the Lhotse Face in that wind. None of us believed them, though. There is no one braver than a Sherpa. We all felt the real reason they were not coming up was that they were spooked by the idea of seeing dead bodies lying all over the Col.

Listening to the wind, we sat in our tents and waited. Hours went by but then the tents became quiet. There was a lull in the wind. Our ears rested until the silence was broken by the buzzing noise of airplanes. They were on the other side of the clouds but no less intrusive because we couldn't see them. Airplanes had no practical reason for being here, so it suddenly struck me that this must be a big news story and the planes were trying to take pictures of a life-and-death struggle. Our tight drama was being invaded by the outside world. It made me angry: If you can't help, then don't come to watch.

Todd and Pete made it to the Col and described a scene of torn tents and gear strewn everywhere. On the way up, at the Geneva Spur, just below Camp IV, they had crossed the Scott Fischer team being led down by guide Neal Beidleman. Some were on oxygen, most were frostbitten, and all were exhausted but they were all moving on their own. Painfully missing from the group was Scott himself— whereabouts unknown—and also Anatoli, who refused to leave the Col without Scott.

Todd and Pete also reported that as they entered Camp IV, Sherpas were leaving from the other side, starting up toward the southeast ridge. They assumed they were trying to reach Rob and Doug. Other Sherpas were also out looking for survivors. Huddled in tents were the remnants of the New Zealand expedition, many too weak to boil water or put oxygen masks on their faces.

The members had little information to offer, most of them unaware even of who was in the tent next to them. Stuart Hutchison did report that Yasuko and Beck were dead. He and a Sherpa had gone out in the morning and found them lying in the snow on the Col about a half mile from camp. They had apparently gotten lost in the white-out. Andy Harris was still nowhere to be found. I was relieved to hear that Frank was back safely. I thought I had killed him by forcing him to stay for that team photo.

Based on Todd's and Pete's assessments, we concluded that none of the survivors was hypothermic and no one was in immediate danger of pulmonary or cerebral edema. They were exhausted and dispirited. The danger of having them descend Lhotse in that condition had to be weighed against the risk of further deterioration at twenty-six thousand feet. On balance, it seemed safer to have everyone spend another night there to rest, eat, drink, and mentally refocus. Todd and Pete continued their work of melting snow, serving food, fluids, and oxygen, and generally trying to be the perfect hosts, though Camp IV wasn't exactly a health spa.

Meanwhile those of us at Camp III turned our attention to the string of ragtag climbers who were descending the fixed lines and would soon be upon us. Members of the IMAX team came up from II to bring supplies and help us out. We set up a kind of waystation at one of their tents—a place to warm up, hydrate, and take a short rest—but Camp III was no place for them to stay. I had almost no medications here, and anyone who needed to lie down would have to be tied in at the 45-degree angle of Lhotse. So everyone had to continue down the ropes to II.

I watched from my tent as the climbers came by one by one. They were moving slowly but none was uncoordinated or in acute distress. Jim hung out on a line below me, acting as official greeter. We dispensed dexamethasone pills to those who looked like they needed it, especially Sandy, who was the most exhausted of the exhausted, then Jim directed each of them to the IMAX tent for food, oxygen, and further encouragement.

Araceli was there, along with some others, smiling as broadly as she could while serving hot tea and soup. As soon as energy and spirits seemed high enough to continue the descent safely, the climbers were sent on their way. No one was allowed to rest too long for fear they would be unable to get going again.

Once our guests were all gone we boiled some water for ourselves and shared a piece of cheese and some chocolate chip cookies. It was pretty meager, so Charles went out to raid the New Zealand tents nearby. He came back with a good haul of food, fuel, and toilet paper. They wouldn't be needing the supplies here anymore and we certainly could use them. Still, it seemed almost ghoulish to be helping ourselves to their supplies while they were in such dire straits.

In quick succession the temperature dropped, it started to snow, and the winds came back—even stronger than before. It had to be much colder and windier higher up and I was beginning to doubt the wisdom of leaving the New Zealand team on the Col another day. Todd reported in to tell us how they were faring.

All the Sherpas had gotten back to IV. Two of them had found Makalu and Scott lying not far from each other. Makalu was still breathing and they dragged him back to camp. Scott was dead.

Anatoli had remained at Camp IV because he didn't want to leave without Scott. Yesterday he had gone out in the blizzard and rescued three climbers. Now with the weather deteriorating rapidly he wanted to go out again to get Scott. It was all Todd and Pete could do to keep him in the camp.

The Sherpas that Todd and Pete had seen leaving camp had tried to go up the southeast ridge. Led by Ang Dorje, Rob's chief climbing Sherpa, they fought their way up but finally were stopped short of the South Summit by the ferocious winds. In the desperate hope that the two stranded climbers could still descend, they left a deposit of oxygen marked with a ski pole at the highest point they had reached. Somewhere, too far above them, were Rob and Doug.

Ang Dorje had just risked his life by climbing a knife-edged ridge buffeted by violent winds to try to save his dying friend, Rob. He cried when he had to turn around. This was the same person who, a week ago at base camp, hadn't shown up to have his tooth pulled because he was too afraid.

We hadn't yet gotten over that radio call before we received another one. Todd said, "You won't believe this. Beck is alive—but I don't know for how long."

Todd had chanced to look out his tent and saw an apparition in the swirling wind and snow. At first he thought it was one of the climbers from camp trying to go to the bathroom, but as he went out to help he realized what it really was: Beck Weathers, risen from the dead.

"His arm was locked straight out from the shoulder, his forearm dangling from his elbow. He looked like a mummy in a low-budget horror flick. He was staggering toward me, into a freezing sixty-mile-an-hour wind, with his jacket open and no glove on his hand."

Todd brought Beck into a tent and put him inside two sleeping bags. But sleeping bags only retain heat, they don't produce it. A hypothermic person can't generate enough heat to keep himself warm so Todd and Pete placed bottles of hot water inside the bags as fast as they could melt snow. They put him on high-flow oxygen and got him to drink some hot liquids. They were doing all the right things by the time they called me.

Rewarming can be tricky and deadly. We didn't want Beck to survive being frozen only to die from being defrosted. It's got to be done evenly and steadily so that there are no sudden shocks which might cause cold-sensitized heart muscles that normally beat synchronously to start contracting independently. The most effective way to transfer a large amount of heat quickly to Beck would have been to take off all his wet clothes and then have either Todd or Pete strip down and get in the sleeping bag with him. Body heat would provide a constant source of warmth radiating over a large surface. I was about to suggest this when Todd told me Beck was coming around.

Todd said Beck's hands were frozen up to his elbows, but there was nothing we could do about that now. There wasn't enough fuel at Camp IV to make enough hot water to thaw Beck's hands. Plus I wasn't sure just how hypothermic Beck still was. If circulation started up in his hands again, the blood that was trapped in there would flow out like a cold wave. When it reached the heart it might be just the shock he didn't need.

We didn't know if Beck's feet were frozen but we didn't want to find out. Taking his boots off would allow his feet to swell, which they were no doubt ready to do if given the chance. It would then be impossible to get them back in the boots, and Beck's only chance of getting down from Camp IV was on his feet, frozen or not. But first he'd have to survive the night on the Col.

Scott, like Beck, had also been pronounced dead, but he was still out there lying in the snow. Anatoli had barely been talked out of going to look for him earlier but now that Beck had returned from the dead, there was no stopping Anatoli as he headed out into the storm. Hours later he came back, alone. He had found Scott but there was no second miracle.

Rob also was out there but much higher up on the southeast ridge. His terrible ordeal came through the radio when we called our base camp to get any news that had been relayed from his base camp. Rob was still in radio contact but his voice was getting weaker and weaker. He said he was below the Hillary Step now and had crawled into a snow cave for shelter. It was unclear what had happened to Doug but Rob seemed to be by himself. Doug had probably died higher up, rather than Rob abandoning him. Earlier he had gotten the message from Todd and Pete, as well as from several others, to leave Doug and try to save himself. His response was, "We're both listening."

So now, except for his radio, Rob was alone. Climbers at base camp urged him to get up and get going and he said okay, he would try. He shut off his radio to conserve the battery and everyone waited hopefully through the silence. A few hours later he turned it back on.

"Where are you now, Rob?"

"You know, I haven't even moved."

Todd and Pete radioed to base camp the unhappy message that Ang Dorje and his team had turned around. The bad news was relayed to Rob: The Sherpas were not going to be able to get him. There was no outburst over the radio. Rob just quietly said, "Okay."

Desperate to get Rob going, the New Zealand base camp manager, Helen Wilton, thought maybe Rob's wife could give him some strength. She patched into the satellite telephone system, then held the phone to the radio as Jan, seven months pregnant, at their home in New Zealand, talked directly to Rob, freezing to death near the summit of Mount Everest. I couldn't even dare to imagine the combination of shock, disbelief, horror, helplessness, and hope that made up their last conversation. Jan tried her best to give him courage and then Rob, incredibly, did the same for her. They chose a name for their baby and he told her not to worry. Finally Rob said he was shutting off his radio so he "can rest." It never came on again.

The storm blew through a second night. Wind speed accelerated to a ferocity I had never experienced before, then got stronger. The wind struck from different directions and our tents, caught in the cross fire, jerked wildly up and down, straining at the ropes, trying to break free of the ice screws that held us against the slope. Any second, we thought, the tents would rip apart or pull out their moorings and we would tumble down the Lhotse Face. We stayed fully dressed with our boots on, spreading out over the floor as much as possible to hold the tent down.

In the morning we were still there but we were grimly aware that it was impossible for Rob to have endured the same night much higher up the mountain and fully exposed. Even now, it was bitter cold and the wind was still strong, though it had relented enough to stop torturing our tents. Lying in our sleeping bags, Steve and I called out almost jokingly to Jim and Charles in the other tent: "Hey, you guys still there?"

There was no response, even after a second try. Suddenly there was real fear that they had been blown off the mountain. A third, louder call brought a somewhat muffled answer. A wall of snow had blown into the narrow space between our tents, insulating the sound. It blocked our entrance but we didn't remove it right away since it also provided some insulation against the cold.

Once more the scene at Camp IV entered our tent through the radio. Beck had survived the night. He was conscious and able to take fluids if Todd or Pete held the cup but he couldn't use his hands and was having trouble seeing. Makalu was also still alive, having been cared for mostly by the Sherpas who had found him. His condition was apparently better than Beck's but only slightly. And there was still no sign of Andy. What was left of the New Zealand team had already started down, all of them under their own power. The Sherpas would shortly be trying to take Makalu down, and Todd and Pete were going to try to bring Beck. Andy, Yasuko, Doug, Rob, and Scott would be staying on the mountain.

Our team was holding at III for the moment. The remnants of the New Zealand team would be passing by soon and might need some help. Makalu and Beck were not yet underway, and being the only doctor on the mountain, I wanted to stay high up in case one or both of them collapsed along the route. The supplies which I had asked for yesterday were waiting for me at Camp II. As soon as we were sure the injured climbers could get all the way down, I would descend to set up a medical tent and wait for my patients.

Pete and Todd were preparing Beck and themselves for the descent. I asked Pete to give Beck some dexamethasone now and to keep some more ready in case he needed it on the road. Pete heated two ampules until they melted and warmed. He injected Beck with one and saved the other inside his jacket. Beck could walk but he couldn't hold the ropes and could barely even see them. The three started off down the slope with Pete in the lead as seeing-eye dog. Beck was in the middle so he could lean his arms against Pete's back, while Todd was behind so he could hold Beck's harness to prevent any fall. Bunched in a tight row and trying to move simultaneously, Beck said, "What is this, a conga line?"

That sounded pretty good. Besides being funny, it meant that Beck was lucid and that, thanks to the exhausting efforts of Pete and Todd, they were probably moving well. The New Zealand team had already passed by us, with Jim once more hanging down from his tent on a rope offering hot tea and oxygen. Business was good and I told him he should consider opening a full-service inn. Once I heard that Makalu was also moving better than expected, and in fact was ahead of Beck, I figured it was time for me to leave.

Jim and I started for Camp II at the same time that Dave and Ed from the IMAX team were moving in the other direction to relieve Todd and Pete and bring Beck the rest of the way. We got down in good time. Just in front of the moraine was an isolated tent that hadn't been there before. It was on the ice, apart from the rest of the Taiwanese camp. We all knew what it was but moved past it without comment. At least Yu Nan had a tent. Five others were still lying in the snow.

Skipping by my own camp I burst into the New Zealand mess tent, coming directly from the Lhotse Face and looking it. The survivors had arrived a while ago and the scene was calm until I entered. Between hugs, handshakes, and pats on the shoulder, I started asking questions and hearing about everyone's injuries at once. There was one person whom I didn't recognize and he was looking at me oddly. He turned out to be a Danish doctor, Henrik Hansen, who had come up from base camp to help out. He reassured me the injuries here were minor, everything was under control, and I should have some tea. I hadn't even sat down yet.

The arrival of two critically ill climbers was imminent. They belonged in a modern hospital intensive care unit but soon I would be treating them here, in a mess tent, trying to work out complex medical problems at an altitude where tying your shoes can be confusing. With Henrik's help plus the help of Sherpas and a few climbers who still had some energy left, we cleared the folding tables and chairs out of the room and covered the floor with foam mats and sleeping bags. Climbers went out to their tents to gather together two complete sets of dry clothes. Sherpas were asked to boil up large pots of water and collect all the insulated bottles they could find. I took an inventory of available supplies and was pleased to see that everything on my list had been brought up that morning, including the heavy propane heater. The Sherpa who carried that up the icefall is one of many unsung heroes.

Frostbite, hypothermia, snow blindness, pulmonary and cerebral edema, pneumonia, dehydration, exhaustion . . . I formed a list in my mind of all the problems I might be dealing with in just a few minutes. For each, I visualized in detail the scenario of what had to be done in what order. Then I systematically laid out medications, bandages, and oxygen bottles, presetting the regulators for maximum flow. I verified that my medical instruments hadn't been damaged or frozen on the trip up.

Only the IV bags were frozen. I passed them out to the Sherpas who were boiling water in the kitchen tent. They brought the bags back twice before they felt warm enough when I touched them to my cheek. Two bags were hung from carabiners that had been hooked into the tent frame. Tubing was connected to each IV and the lines were flushed. The loose ends of the tubes were left dangling above the still-empty sleeping bags. Everything seemed to be working. I felt entirely ready.

By radio we were kept advised of my patients' progress. Makalu was already down off the ropes and Beck wasn't far behind. We turned on the propane heater and I instructed the Sherpas to start bringing in the tubs of hot water from the kitchen. Lopsang took advantage of the opportunity to draw off some of the water to serve tea.

In the oddly quiet interlude, we sipped and waited just long enough for my mind to start wandering. Suddenly, there was a commotion outside, the tent door was unzipped and in strode a bulky creature in a hooded down suit with an oxygen mask over his face, escorted by a group of Sherpas. As ready as I was, his appearance took me by surprise and for a split second I said to myself, "What is that?"

It was Makalu of course. We immediately laid him down on a sleeping bag and started taking off his clothes; jacket after jacket, layer after layer. His rescuers had bundled him up in anything they could find. His clothes were all wet, including his underwear. Getting his boots off was difficult since his feet had swelled tightly against them. If they expanded any more, we'd have to find a larger pair of boots to put back on him later. I had to use a scalpel to cut away part of a sock which had frozen to his foot. I left it to the Sherpas to maneuver around me and work a set of dry clothes onto him while I started my examination.

When I removed his oxygen mask, I was shocked. Makalu, the climber who seemed indifferent to his partner's death, was the climber who had kindly shared his water with me when I passed him on the Lhotse ropes—except that now he was missing his nose. Instead, there was a black crust that spread onto his right cheek up to his eye. He probably had some snow blindness but his eyes were puffed closed so tightly that I couldn't tell for sure.

"My eyes, my face, all was ice," he told me. "My hands together—*clink, clink.*"

Makalu had the worst frostbite I had ever seen. All the fingers on both hands were dark gray, plump like sausages. The color extended onto the hands to form a sharply demarcated gray band across the knuckles. There were strong pulses in each wrist, indicating that blood was flowing into the hands, at least up to the gray line. His feet had the same gray color from the toes onto the forefoot, as well as across the heels. I found pulses in his ankles and marked them with a pen so that I could check later to see if they were still there.

The frostbite was probably irreversible, but if we could thaw him out, parts of his hands and feet could be saved. Once thawed, he'd have to be kept warm. When limbs thaw, blood vessels break and surrounding tissue weakens, making it less able to withstand a second onslaught. Any part that refroze would be worse off than if it had never defrosted. His thawed-out feet would be fragile. If he were allowed to bear weight on them, they'd crumble. At twenty-one thousand feet the treatment problem was all in the logistics but with enough help, enough fuel, and more than enough snow to melt, I thought it could be done.

Henrik had started an IV, using a salt solution with glucose to provide fluids and energy. I injected nifedipine to divert blood into the extremities. This would begin to improve circulation in the hands and feet, but the diminished volume in the center of the body could lead to a rapid drop in blood pressure. Having no pressure cuff, the only way to monitor him was by periodically feeling the strength of the carotid artery pulsations in his neck. Any sudden weakening might mean he was going into shock. If that happened, we'd try to counteract it by opening wide the IV valve to pump him back up with fluids.

We needed three tubs of warm water—one for each hand and one for the feet. By trial and error we got Makalu positioned so that all his frozen parts could be submerged at the same time. I had a deck of little plastic bubble thermometer cards and dropped one in each tub. Maintaining an ideal defrosting temperature of 104 degrees is a lot of work when the ambient temperature is below zero. The water cools rapidly and has to be canted off so hot water can be added. The Sherpas were eager assistants and quickly got the hang of it, using cups to remove the water and insulated bottles to add more. Most of them had never used a thermometer before, but soon they were reading the temperatures and making their own decisions on when to add water.

Just as we were getting Makalu under control, we got word that Beck was about to arrive. It was time to put dressings on Makalu anyway. The rewarming had no real end point, and getting him waterlogged wouldn't help. My supplies were limited so I had to parcel them out carefully. Beck was reportedly worse off than Makalu but Makalu's condition was plenty bad enough. I decided to divide my supplies in half. After patting dry Makalu's hands and feet, I put on gooey ointment and antibiotic dressings, separating fingers and toes with thin gauze so they wouldn't stick together. Then I wrapped the hands and feet with fluffy cotton dressings which were far too bulky to fit in gloves or socks, so I covered them with down booties to keep them warm. Makalu was tucked into his sleeping bag and pushed to one side to make room for the next customer.

Beck was helped in by Ed and Dave, who had taken the relay from Todd and Pete above Camp III. I was expecting an incoherent, half-blind, semiconscious phantom but, as he was being eased to the floor, he said to me in an easy, conversational tone, "Hi, Ken, where should I sit?"

Ed and Dave and I shook hands and congratulated one another on the great job we were doing. Then they left to let us do our work. Beck was alert and coordinated, showing no signs of hypothermia. Edema, though, had swollen his face to twice its size. I hardly recognized him. His cheeks were black and his nose had burned down to a piece of charcoal. I was afraid if he sneezed, he would blow it away.

Makalu had had the worst frostbite I had ever seen, but that was before I saw Beck. His entire right hand and a third of his forearm, as well as his entire left hand, were deep purple and frozen solid. They radiated cold. There were no blisters, no pulses, no sensation, no pain. They were the hands of a dead man, but bizarrely, he could move his fingers since the live muscles in his forearm, like the strings of a marionette, were able to pull on the dead bones in his hand.

His eyesight was better than I expected, with no evidence of snow blindness. The loss of vision had been due to the aftereffects of eye surgery. He had had a radial keratotomy to correct his sight, but the operation leaves scars on the corneas. At high altitude his corneas swelled, but the scars made the expansion uneven, causing blurry images. Now with the decrease in altitude, his eyes were curing themselves.

We went through the same routine with Beck as we had for Makalu except that frostbite had only barely touched his toes, so a third tub for soaking his feet wasn't needed. The Sherpas were now masters of rewarming but even with only two tubs to maintain, they were having difficulty keeping up. For all practical purposes, Beck's hands were blocks of ice and they cooled the water too rapidly.

As we worked, Beck talked casually. Anyone hearing the conversation without seeing what was going on would have thought he had just dropped by for tea. He told me his vision had progressively deteriorated on summit day and by the time he reached the southeast ridge he was unable to see well enough to start along that narrow edge. Because Rob didn't want him descending alone, he told him to wait there and he'd pick him up on the way back from the summit. That didn't happen and so Beck finally started down late with another group of climbers. He had just gotten off the triangular face onto the South Col when the storm came up. With the fog and wind-driven snow, visibility quickly went to zero and he became separated from the others. Since the South Col is flat and featureless, he was unable to find his way back to camp. Wandering around in the bitter wind and cold he realized his hands were numb so he decided to take his gloves off to put his hands inside his jacket. He got his right glove off and opened the jacket but the wind blew the glove away and he was never able to get his hand inside. Lost and exhausted, he collapsed in the snow.

He said he was in a timeless, dreamlike state, not unconscious, but unable to move. He became aware of someone bending over him, saying, "He's dead." In fact, he had been lying in the snow overnight and by morning he realized he wasn't dead but if he didn't do something he soon would be. He summoned up all his courage and all his strength, and stood up. He was able to reason that since the wind had been behind him when he started out, he'd have to face into it to get back. He staggered ahead through the whiteout until he became the apparition Todd saw outside his tent.

Beck told me the story quietly and casually but I was struck by the power of what he had done. Out of oxygen, exhausted, and hypothermic, he had been able to rally his mind enough to get his body moving and focus his thoughts. He had transcended the laws of medicine. The only way to explain it was that it was a miracle.

It was time to wrap up Beck's hands. As I was preparing the bandages, Charles came in for the third time. He had been acting as my mother hen, making roundtrips from our camp to bring me food, which I didn't eat, then later to bring me warmer clothes as it got colder. This trip he brought me my sleeping bag and toothbrush, as it had become obvious I wasn't going back to our camp any time soon. He was eager to help, so I had him assist me in applying the dressings. I knew he would be thrilled to participate in the medical treatment. Charles spread the fingers, positioning the hand precisely as I asked, and Beck's hands were soon wrapped like Makalu's. Since all my dressings were now gone, I gave Charles a list of supplies to have sent up from base camp for use the next day, in case we couldn't evacuate these guys.

For most of the New Zealand climbers, fatigue had overcome excitement but a few climbers were still hanging around, including one who had relatively minor frostbite. His hand had been wrapped earlier but he had gone to the bathroom since then and now the bandage was grossly contaminated. Patiently he waited for me to finish, then asked if I could change his dressing. All I could offer him was sympathy. I had nothing left to rewrap him with, nor even any good advice on where he could put his hand.

Frank hadn't left yet either. There was a camera around and he was a professional photographer so, after checking with Makalu and Beck, I asked him to take some pictures. I'm sure the thought occurred to him a lot earlier, but his sense of propriety prevented him from even suggesting it. Once I turned him loose, he set about his work diligently until the camera got stuck, probably from the cold.

Even though Frank looked really tired and wasn't taking pictures anymore, he didn't want to leave yet. I sensed he wanted some attention but he was afraid to ask for it, seeing the severity of the injuries around him. Things were quiet now so I sat down next to him and asked how he was feeling. He was quick to respond, asking if I could just look at his feet to be sure he didn't have frostbite. I took a good, serious look, then reassured him that he didn't. That seemed to be just what he needed. He was in better shape than any of the others because he had been the first to turn around. He said the two best sights were Todd coming into his tent at Camp IV and me coming into his tent at Camp II. I wanted to ask him what happened up there, but this wasn't the time or place.

As I was watching my patients, a pretty Japanese woman knelt beside Makalu and, speaking softly, encouraged him to sip from the bowl of soup she was holding. I was pleased that she was taking it upon herself to feed the patients and make them comfortable, considerations to which doctors often don't give enough importance. As she rearranged the mat Beck was lying on, I realized that she was Sumiyo, the IMAX starlet.

Makalu and Beck were stabilized although their conditions were fragile and could worsen suddenly. I was anxious to get them out of here. Base camp had some surprising news for us: A high-performance military helicopter was on alert. If winds were calm in the morning, it would attempt to land at Camp I, avoiding the need to make the treacherous descent through the icefall. At nineteen thousand feet, it would probably be the highest helicopter rescue ever. Pilots had never before been willing to come above base camp. We speculated that this story must be getting big publicity and the Nepalese wanted to try to pull off something spectacular.

Meanwhile, at Camp II, we were in a freezing tent getting colder by the minute. Our only propane heater, aimed directly on Beck and Makalu, did nothing for the rest of us or for the IV bags hanging from the top of the tent. Warm fluids had to keep flowing into our patients. We'd make them hypothermic if the bags got even half as cold as we were. While Henrik and I were discussing the problem, Sumiyo nodded her head and left. A few minutes later she came back and put the solution in our hands—a bunch of chemical hand warmers that we promptly activated and tied around the IV bags.

One by one everyone settled into their sleeping bags except me. Even though I had spent last night holding my tent down, and this morning had made a descent from Lhotse, I was still in overdrive and knew I wouldn't be able to sleep. I out-volunteered Henrik to keep watch, promising to wake him if I got tired. In the cold, silent tent I watched the IV fluids drip and the oxygen tank gauges gradually lose their pressure. I listened to the rhythmic breathing of my patients, periodically took their pulses, and added drops to Makalu's eyes whenever he complained of pain. I could feel the air temperature drop degree by degree as surely as if I had a thermometer to measure it. As much as possible I tried to work from inside my sleeping bag, but my feet were freezing despite putting heavy mitts over my socks and wrapping them in a down jacket. I would have felt guilty turning the propane heater toward myself, so I just stayed cold and had a miserable night.

At about four o'clock Henrik awoke by himself, but I stayed up anyway, by now too cold and too tired to fall asleep. I felt terrible but I didn't dare think about it, knowing what others had been through. Deciding to be optimistic, Henrick and I began to get Beck and Makalu ready for a helicopter ride. It was slow work. I could hardly get myself going, much less them. Progress was minimal until we woke up the Sherpas who took over most of the work and even made us tea.

An hour before dawn we got the discouraging word from base camp that it was too windy. The helicopter wasn't coming. I had to make a hard decision. We could try to wait out the wind, but it might stay windy for days. At this altitude even a minor cut couldn't heal, and with the injuries they suffered, Beck and Makalu would rapidly deteriorate. Taking them down through the icefall, though, would expose them to further cold and trauma, not to mention the risk to the rescuers who would be transporting them beneath ice walls and through crevasse fields. Climbers are always willing to risk their lives to save others. Knowing that my decision would be carried out without question made the responsibility weigh even heavier, but the needs of my two patients were compelling. I opted for the over-the-ice evacuation.

As the patients were being fed, dressed, and tended to, I discreetly redirected the heater to thaw out my feet. Once I could feel them, I walked over to let Todd know the helicopter wasn't coming and we'd have to do it the hard way. Immediately, Todd began to organize rescue teams and I went back to finish packing up Beck and Makalu. I pulled out their IVs and disconnected them from the oxygen tanks. With the oxygen masks removed, I was able for the first time to treat their frostbitten faces with a burn cream. As I applied the white pasty cream to Beck's nose and cheeks, I remarked that I was putting on makeup so he'd look good at base camp.

The escorts arrived. Since Beck could walk, Todd and Pete led him out and started down the Cwm. Makalu's feet were frostbitten; he had to be carried. The Sherpas, experts at carrying loads, tied him to an aluminum frame and then mounted it to a harness on the back of the first volunteer. They would have to take turns carrying and dragging this unusually heavy load.

The parade stretched out down the Cwm, with Jim and me bringing up the rear. Progress was slow but this was the "easy" part. The difficulties and the dangers would soon increase dramatically as we entered the icefall. I was entirely preoccupied with how the trip would affect Makalu and Beck and how I would manage them at base camp. Methodically following Jim's footsteps, I was barely aware of the surroundings. My enclosed space was disrupted, however, by a noisy green insect coming at us from out of the sky. It startled me back to the present.

The wind had died down and the helicopter was going to try to land. It circled once and came in low, testing the air to see if there was enough of it. The rotor wash, bouncing the air back up off the surface, gave the helicopter some extra lift but the effect was lost when it passed over a deep crevasse. The tail suddenly dropped and swung forward, nearly catching in the ice. The pilot was looking for a landing spot but from the air, hidden crevasses are hard to see. They are hard enough to see even from the ground. Ed picked out a spot that looked safe but had nothing with which to mark it until Araceli tossed him a bottle of red Kool-Aid she was carrying. He used it to mark a big X for a landing pad and then tied a bandanna to a ski pole to make a wind sock. The pilot came straight down but only lightly touched the ice, aware that if the skids got stuck and he couldn't take off, he'd be unable to survive at this altitude.

The pilot held up a single finger—there was only enough lift for one passenger. Beck immediately deferred to Makalu. He knew that because Makalu had to be carried, his trip through the icefall would be the more hazardous one for all involved. He also knew that the pilot might not be able to land a second time.

As the helicopter disappeared, Beck asked Pete if he thought it would be back. Pete replied, "You'll be in time for brunch at the Yak and Yeti Hotel."

The pilot ferried Makalu over the icefall to base camp and then came back for Beck, who boarded with a cry of joy. The helicopter disappeared for the second and final time from the Cwm. In the thicker air at base camp, Makalu was put back on board with Beck. They would both be in Kathmandu before we were out of the icefall. Ahead of us was merely another "routine" descent to base camp. There was a huge sense of relief and pride which we all shared, but I also felt an intense letdown, a sudden sense of disengagement. A challenge far greater than summiting had been removed and the exhilaration that came from rising to it was left hanging in the air behind the helicopter.

CHAPTER
13

The base camp we had left with high hopes so long ago was gone. What we returned to was a forlorn group of tents pitched on a glacier. There were a lot of hugs but not much talking. We all knew what we were feeling and conversation would have been redundant. The camps were inhabited by energyless climbers and more than a few zombies. Gestures like smiling or saying hello seemed superfluous so we often walked past each other without any acknowledgement. The absence of a handful of climbers made all the camps feel empty.

It was cold out, but I was colder. The chill from my night at Camp II was still with me and the air seemed to penetrate no matter what I wore. My heaviest set of thermal underwear was rolled into a ball in the corner of my tent. Last week I had switched to cleaner ones for my summit attempt, but now the others appeared cleaner than what I was wearing. I was too lethargic even to think about doing a wash so after reconsideration, I decided that the ones in the corner weren't too dirty to put back on.

Apparently some people were even colder and more lethargic than I was. A climber came to ask if I had any extra thermal underwear. I held up what I had: "I just took this set off because it's too dirty, but it's warm."

"That's fine. I'll take it," she said.

Those with the most serious injuries had either been evacuated or were still lying on the mountain, but there were lots of climbers with less-severe injuries walking around base camp. Our medical tent was well stocked and became a self-serve dispensary for anyone who needed a dressing change. I was available as technical adviser for those who didn't feel comfortable as do-it-yourselfers.

Ingrid came by to pick up some supplies. On summit day she had been holding a radio when her camp got the news about Scott. She threw the radio up in the air and let it smash on the rocks. She was still in pretty fragile shape. She couldn't ask me where the gauze pads were without crying.

A vent was needed. The anger, grief, and frustration had to be released and shared. Scott's group passed the word that they were going to hold a memorial service at their camp. Everyone was invited to come and listen and say whatever they felt like.

The gray, overcast sky matched the somber mood of the climbers who gathered together that afternoon. Some stood and some sat on the cold rocks, forming a circle in front of the lhapso fire. Almost everyone was connected to someone else by a hand, an arm, or a shoulder, for emotional support as well as for warmth in the chilly air. Two Sherpas sat with their knees folded under them, facing the altar. Their prayer book, a stack of parchments laced together by yak hide, rested before them on an oxygen crate. We were enveloped by a mesmerizing mixture of juniper smoke and monotone chanting.

As the music continued on, a woman with her face and hands bandaged came out of Scott's group and, using two ski poles as crutches, walked up to the high rocks near the altar. She said, "My name is Charlotte and I'd like to recite a poem." That broke the ice and she was followed by one speaker after another who, simply and spontaneously, said what they felt.

"Scott Fischer . . . on summit day he said he wasn't feeling so good—but Scott was Scott and I knew he'd be okay . . ."

"Rob Hall . . . the most respected high altitude mountaineer in the world. He refused to abandon a dying climber. I would have expected no less from him . . ."

"Andy Harris . . . I thought he was back safely but in the whiteout he missed the camp by a few yards and stepped off the East Face . . ."

"Doug Hansen . . . in our tent he showed me pictures of his daughter. Let's never forget that other people have a precious investment in us that we have to protect . . ."

"Yasuko Namba . . . I was trying to drag her and two others to safety. I felt her slip off and I let her go. I didn't have the strength to hold her any longer . . ."

Occasionally one of the speakers would turn toward the mountain to speak from the heart directly to one of the climbers still up there. It occurred to me that Beck Weathers had died up there too. But he was the only one who had been brought back to life.

The Sherpas had finished their chanting, but people were still stepping up to speak until finally, there was no movement. In the long silence it seemed that everyone who wanted a turn had taken it. Then Lopsang, the sirdar for Scott's team stood up. He had left Scott on the Southeast Ridge only after Scott collapsed and threatened to jump off it if Lopsang didn't descend alone to save himself. Now, with his head down, Lopsang started to cry and said, "I tried and I tried and I tried but I couldn't save him."

No one could save them. The people next to Lopsang put their arms around him and then around each other, releasing the emotion in all of us. There were tears and tight hugs as everyone tried to console everyone else, and themselves.

Finally, Neal said, "If no one else wants to speak, that's it. But we'll be here a couple more days and if you want to talk, please come by and have a cup of coffee on Scott."

The wind was picking up, snapping the prayer flags that were strung from the lhapso. The Sherpas believe that if you write prayers on the flags, the wind will carry the messages up to the gods. But I guess this year Everest wasn't listening. I threw some rice on the fire and walked away.

So where was Rob?, I thought to myself the next morning, still not fully awake. The memorial service was an important event. He should have been there. My head cleared: We had been friends for ten years. It was hard to imagine Everest without him.

Having decompressed at the service, we all now had room to think about, and talk about, what happened up there. It was time to talk to Frank. He had gone with the New Zealand team this year because it was his fifth trip to Everest and he wanted to change his luck. He did, but not in the way he expected.

Frank said that because of a strong wind, they had gotten to the Col late and hardly had any rest. All they got to eat was half a bowl of warm water. Everyone was tired and running on empty. The winds picked up that evening and blew constantly. Frank said he prayed that they wouldn't go for the summit that night; that the high winds would make them take a rest day. But just before midnight the winds calmed and Rob decided to go for it. Frank thought the decision was forced because there wasn't enough oxygen to stay another day at the Col. Shortly after they started, it turned bitter cold and the winds picked up again. Frank was the first to drop out. It took courage to say, "This is not for me," and turn around while everyone else was pressing on. That decision saved his life and maybe also the life of someone else who would have tried to rescue him.

Frank was leaving today. He had come in with two bags but was going out with one. He gave all his climbing gear to the Sherpas. He said he would never climb again.

A lot of people were leaving the mountain as fast as they could, some no doubt carrying away the same sentiments as Frank. Those who remained from Scott's and Rob's camps were invited by us to dinner one night and we all fit easily in our mess tent.

There was only one topic of conversation. Neal said he couldn't understand how someone like Scott, who had climbed Everest once before without oxygen, wasn't able to make it down this time even with it. Pete voiced the consensus that Rob had violated his own rule about a strict turnaround time. Jim thought that maybe after seeing Scott's team summit, Rob was overanxious to get his people up. We recalled that last year too, Rob had cut his safety margin thin on summit day and barely got everyone back. . . . That year there had been no storm.

Pete, Jim, and I and six others had gone for the summit last year, two days after Rob's team. We encountered the same conditions but turned back much sooner, though we were only nine hundred feet below the top. I couldn't help thinking that had we persisted that day, this disaster would have been about us.

I was asked how I could explain Beck's survival. As a doctor, I had to say that being hypothermic is like being in hibernation. You can't be sure that someone is cold and dead until he is first warm and dead. But what I really thought was—you can't explain it. A miracle is something that just happens. Then humans cobble together an explanation for it because they feel more comfortable when they think they understand. It's too unsettling to confront the unknown.

Todd thought it was time to lighten the discussion. My face had gotten badly burned those last few days on the mountain so he said, "Ken, you're so dark you should eat in the Sherpa kitchen."

I said, "Can you imagine how much darker I'll get if I start eating their dahlbat?"

It didn't bring much of a laugh. Other climbers tried to liven up the group. Despite the females present, or maybe because of them, they told dirty jokes. Nothing sounded very funny but we laughed anyway.

Later, after our guests from the two disastrous expeditions had left, it seemed the time was right to discuss whether we should try again for the summit. Charles pointed out that "again" is inappropriate since "we haven't even tried once." Steve asked, "If we leave like this, what did we come here for?"—a good question that had recently gotten a lot harder to answer no matter how we left.

It was apparent that each of us had already worked through an answer, but discussing another attempt too soon would have trivialized the loss of our friends, and planning for it would almost be like pretending the disaster never happened. The idea of returning to the mountain would be unthinkable to the outside world. It would be seen as blatant, incomprehensible stupidity, and if someone else got hurt, it would be indefensible. Yet we were unanimous in wanting to go back up.

How could we, after seeing our friends die? These deaths at this time were shocking, to be sure, but death on the mountain is no surprise. We had long since come to accept the risk, otherwise we wouldn't have been here in the first place. A demonstration of the risk, though dramatic and horrifying, didn't cause us to waiver from our previous assessment. Had the accident revealed a danger that we were unaware of, we would have recalculated the odds, but the already known risks of sudden storm, hypothermia, and exhaustion weren't reasons to stop our expedition now if they weren't reasons before. We couldn't pretend though, that nothing had changed. The same odds we accepted before seemed more foolhardy now that their impact was real. Risk was no longer an abstract term.

Reality was becoming uncomfortable. I didn't allow myself to think about it, afraid that if I did, I might be inevitably drawn to a sobering conclusion. I wanted to act on a self-centered impulse without the influence of inconvenient facts derived from family responsibility. Uncertain now how I would deal with those facts, I'd rather keep them at a distance. One contact with home and I might lose my insulation.

Coming down from the rescue, I became aware that our mountain drama was playing to the entire world. News of the disaster probably had at least a day's headstart over the message relayed out from our camp that we were all safe. The interval must have been terrifying for my wife and family. Even though I got to base camp after they had been reassured, I knew Josiane would love to hear that message in my own voice. But how reassuring would I be, telling her I was planning to go back up in a few days? And how would I be able to justify the decision if she forced me to look at it rationally? There was a satellite phone in the IMAX tent, but I didn't make the call.

The IMAX tent also had a satellite fax, and every day Dave came over to show us the latest weather map. The jet stream showed no sign of slowing down, so that meant the wind was favorable—for me. I could use a few days of enforced rest. I was still feeling the effect of my night at Camp II and so was Henrik. We listened to each other's lungs once but didn't like what we heard and ignored the other's advice not to climb anymore.

Necessities of doctoring kept intruding on my desire to be listless. There were no other doctors left—Henrik was here only as a climber—but there were still a lot of Sherpas around, so my medical tent continued to be a walk-in clinic.

The wind took a dip and our break was over. The next morning, with no fanfare, we left on our summit attempt. Henrik also was climbing today and he passed me going up the icefall. A few hours later he passed me again on his way down. He said he wasn't moving fast enough and it would be dangerous to attempt Everest like this. What he didn't say was, "Are you crazy to be going up? You're slower than me."

Stubbornly I persisted all the way through the icefall but no one feels better at Camp I than he does at base camp. The expedition was over for me. The next morning, as the rest of the team moved on to Camp II, I dragged myself back down with Nima Tashi as my escort. My motivation for moving as fast as I could wasn't because of the dangers of the unstable ice. I was more afraid that if I moved too slowly, Nima Tashi would try to carry me. What an ignominious end to the expedition that would be.

As he walked me back to my tent, Nima Tashi had tears in his eyes. He was more disappointed than I was. Putting his pack down he took out a paper cylinder containing some pictures. I recognized them as the ones the children had drawn for him to decorate his hospital room after his surgery. He was planning to take them with us to the summit. He really thought we would do it this time. Nima Tashi wanted to say more but was frustrated by his lack of English. There was no need to speak; I could see it all in his face.

It was time for the satellite phone. I had taken my chance and was no longer vulnerable to the inconsistencies in my logic. Josiane was just purely and simply happy to hear from me. She had received word that I was safe before she even knew what it was I was safe from. She hadn't heard about the disaster the day before but did think it was strange that, after I had already been away two months, friends were suddenly, casually, asking her if she heard from Kenny. With the question of survivors still unanswered, no one had wanted to break the potentially fatal news to her.

She told me Jonathan was waiting to have a catch with me and Jennifer said that if I don't get back soon she was going to finish her lanyard without me.

It was time to go home. I had to wait for the rest of the team, but that didn't take too long. After holding a few days at Camp II for the wind to quiet down, they called off the expedition. They had no mental reserves left and lacked the spirit to climb Everest.

There were only a few camps left on the glacier. The place where the New Zealand camp had been was now a pile of rocks. As I walked past it I imagined the tents and the bustling activity that had been here just one week earlier. Healthy, young, vibrant people who were with us then were now high up on Everest frozen in the snow. What a joyful, exuberant place this would be right now if things had gone differently.

The snow was getting too soft, the avalanches were increasing, the outhouse was collapsing, and the ice under my tent was melting. The monsoon was on its way. It was time to go. Maybe it had never been time to come.

I was leaving without answers. If the real goal of a climb is not to get to the top but to return safely, why go at all? What makes a seemingly intelligent person willing to take a risk for a goal with no practical value? Why engage in a pursuit that can only be considered frivolous and selfish when balanced against the impact of a loss of life?

There is no goal that is at the same time more real and more abstract than the top of a mountain. Maybe some of the answers lie therein. A summit is a clearly definable objective that can be reached by dedication, good planning, hard work, and luck. The first look at a big mountain fills you with fear: It's impossibly huge; no human can climb that; no human belongs there. But to control your fear, you think of the mountain as steps, and taking one at a time, you find there is no single step you cannot make. You keep moving upward until every direction leads down and you realize, after a moment's confusion, that you're at the top. There were no impossible obstacles; the only barriers were in your mind.

Mountains are immutable and indifferent; they can't be conquered. What you conquer are your fears and your perceived limitations. Easy challenges are no challenges, but hard ones come with bigger risks. Dealing with those risks will call on dormant strengths in yourself that you might otherwise never have discovered. Nothing is more empowering than taking a risk and succeeding.

We hold in esteem those who take the greater risks but if they lose, do we then call them foolish? Worse, what if they die trying? What a stupid, needless waste of a life.

As a climbing doctor, I've seen much injury and death in the mountains. On Everest there are frozen bodies lying along the route. As I pass them I turn away and block them out of my mind. But now there will be five more, and their images won't be so easy to block out. Saying "they died doing what they loved" doesn't replace the sense of personal loss. The "thrill of the climb" seems pretty thin when measured against the devastation of families.

So why did I come here and why will I come back? Because climbing reduces life to its simplest, most basic elements: food, shelter, survival. Humans are designed to deal with these essentials, not the trivia that fills our everyday modern lives. Climbing elevates the senses to a higher pitch, emotions become intense and, unexpectedly, it's relaxing. Challenging nature on its own basic terms and succeeding brings exhilaration on a grand scale.

I didn't get to the summit. Along the way I had the chance to renounce my personal goal and take part in a noble cause—a medical challenge which tested me as much as the mountain did but, in my heart, pleased me more. I didn't reach the top but I succeeded.

Each of us should have his or her own Everest—a testing place in any endeavor where the goal is almost, but not quite, beyond reach. When you take on a great challenge and persevere, you discover that your abilities are more than you ever imagined, enabling you at times to accomplish the "impossible." A life lived in this way is infinitely fulfilling. It strikes such a responsive chord in so many people that it must resonate with a primitive human instinct.

"If you have a dream, begin it.
Boldness has genius, power, and magic in it."

POSTSCRIPT

The preceding quote is a paraphrase from an eighteenth-century poem by Johann Goethe, popular among climbers who are attracted to big mountains. The sentiment is what brought many of us to Everest. Our lives crossed there briefly and then we moved on, each along his or her own path but none of us unaffected by the mountain.

Lopsang was tormented by the death of Scott Fischer. Four months later he returned to Everest and, while high up on the Lhotse face, was caught in an avalanche that buried him not so far from the friend he didn't want to leave.

Anatoli Boukreev received the American Alpine Club's highest award for his courage during the storm. Anatoli believed there wasn't enough luck in the world, and he used up a lot on Everest. His share ran out Christmas Day one and a half years later on Annapurna when he was swept away by an avalanche.

Beck Weathers lost all of his right hand and most of his left but he responded spectacularly to his second chance at life. He has returned to work as a pathologist, written a book, *Left for Dead,* and is a much sought-after inspirational speaker. Conversations with Beck are always delightfully positive, and I continue to be awed by his indomitable spirit.

Makalu Gau spent almost a year in hospitals, first in the U.S. and then in Taiwan. He lost most of each hand, parts of his feet and his entire nose. Reportedly, he has great difficulty walking but can write and use chopsticks. I lost contact with him when he left Alaska after doctors there tried to fit him with a facial prosthesis. He said he knew then that it was time to go home—he didn't want a Caucasian nose.

Jan Arnold is a single mom in New Zealand, practicing medicine part-time so she can have more time for her daughter, Sarah—the name she and Rob chose together. Sarah is four years old now, and Jan says she has Rob's personality.

Frank Fischbeck lives quietly in Hong Kong, still publishing high-quality books and taking brilliant photographs. He hasn't yet gone back to climbing.

Margo Chisholm never did summit Everest, but she overcame far harder challenges. She told her story in her book, *To the Summit,* and she continues to be an inspiration to those with addiction problems.

Chantal Mauduit lit up climbing routes wherever she went. She became famous in France for her climbing accomplishments and her style. She wasn't on Everest in 1996, but two years later she was on another Himalayan peak, Dhaulagiri, when a small avalanche hit her tent. She was killed in her sleep.

Nima Tashi summited Everest three more times on his fused ankle. He is in high demand for expeditions, and he and his family have prospered. They built a teahouse in Pangboché and decorated the walls with my children's pictures.

It took two more expeditions, one led by Wally Berg and one by Pete Athans, before enough data was accumulated for Brad Washburn to determine the exact height of Everest: 29,035 feet; good news for the Nepalese, since Everest is actually higher, by seven feet, than was previously thought. The king of Nepal was pleased and proud. The height has not changed in at least four years despite enormous tectonic pressure from below. Brad discovered a series of fault lines below the mountain that he expects will yield one day, creating a sudden upthrust. He advised me that if I intend to summit Everest, I should do it soon, before the mountain gets any higher.

I've been back to Everest two more times since the disasters, but not to climb. I served as Chief High Altitude Physician on two research projects sponsored in part by NASA, to field test position locators and remote medical sensing devices that could be used in a space station or on Mars. The space-age sensors were worn by climbers and provided real-time monitoring of their location and physical condition. In a severe storm, the system would indicate where each climber was and whether he or she was alive. If we had had these devices on Everest in 1996, perhaps we could have saved some of the people who never left the mountain.

EPILOGUE

The mist that hung in the back of my mind has cleared. Climbing and I are no longer remote—we've become intimate. Rather than existing in a different life, climbing has intertwined itself in mine. I explored the mountains that appeared out of the mist and the secret places I imagined were converted into reality.

By the time I got to Everest, none of the ice in the icefall I had read about was still there; it had all long since passed into the sea. Yet the icefall remains the same. New ice replaces the old. The icefall flows. It retains its beauty and its essence precisely because it changes. It is constantly renewed.

People's lives flow as well. The time will come when no one who passes the Sherpa memorial will have known anyone whose name is carved on the stones there now. They will behold the place as I first did, and bring no prayer shawls to tie around the monuments. They will discover mountaineering anew but before their adventures are over, some of them will feel the need to place shawls, as I do now, and some of them will be the ones for whom the shawls are placed.

All things in nature must change if they are to retain their vitality. Ideas can live forever, but little boys grow up. They must entrust their ideas to the adults they are to become. What if I were to be confronted by the little boy I was?

He would ask me, "What have you done with my life? Did you fulfill the trust I gave you?" The answer must, of necessity, fall short of his hopes. A child's imagination is unencumbered by reality. An adult has to navigate through the dizzying experiences of life and can't take the straight route the naive child imagines. But was the child's intensity and direction blunted and deflected by real obstacles or did the adult just get lost in the details along the way—always moving but going nowhere? I would answer the little boy, "I held your trust tightly as I was propelled into the world, buffeted and bombarded by forces outside my control. Had I remained unchanged throughout, it would mean life had had no impact on me. What value would it have had then? Why live it? I changed—but I steered as close as I could to the life you imagined for me." In our final accounting, I believe the boy would be satisfied with the man he has become.

Turning from the past, I look at the future. I see my children, about the same age as that little boy—the cycle continues. The impressions they form now will be the most intense of their lives. My mountaineering books are on my shelves, along with my medical books and many others. Whatever books they decide to open, or whatever catches their imagination, I hope it creates a big dream. Encouraging them to pursue that dream will give them purpose and stability, ignite their potential and make them the best they can be. The measure of their success won't be in the destination they pick, but in the journey they make to get there. A life lived with potential fulfilled will bring contentment—the greatest blessing anyone can receive.

As one generation links to the next, children carry the flow of renewal. In years to come, I'll be replaced by offspring who never knew me. I'll be anonymous, but if I can pass along to them the spirit that I found in the mountains, no matter what form it takes, I will have touched eternity.

Having looked at the past and at the future, I see the present more clearly. I've lived a lot of adventures, seen a lot of disasters, and I've been lucky. But reaching the top of a mountain is not nearly as necessary as getting back. My wife and children have a huge investment in me, and I in them. Climbing has brought me contentment on a grand scale, but so has surgery, and especially, so has my home life. Goethe's noble words ring in my ears, but I also hear Josiane's quiet voice reminding me how much I have at home. The family of little stuffed dolls is all together on a shelf. It will be much harder to separate them now.